The Road Back

THE ROAD BACK

Rheumatoid Arthritis: Its Cause and Its Treatment

Thomas McPherson Brown, M.D., and Henry Scammell

M. EVANS AND COMPANY, INC. NEW YORK

Library of Congress Cataloging-in-Publication Data

Brown, Thomas McPherson.
The road back.

Includes index.
1. Rheumatoid arthritis—Popular works. I. Scammell, Henry. II. Title.
RC933.B77 1988 616.7′22 88-3606

ISBN 0-87131-543-2

M. Evans and Company, Inc.
216 East 49 Street
New York, New York 10017

Design by Lauren Dong

Manufactured in the United States of America

9 8 7 6 5 4 3 2 1

Contents

To our wives, Olive and Caroline,
for their faith,

to the volunteers and staff of the Arthritis Institute,
for their support,

to Rob Maguire and Doug Reddan,
for giving the Institute its start and sustenance,

to Jane Fagan,
for everything, especially her introduction,

To Tom Hallowell,
for a lifetime of friendship
and for his financial backing when it counted most,

to all the members of Tom Brown's Army, 10,000 strong,
for their abiding courage,

and particularly to those whose stories are on these pages,
for their generosity,

this book is lovingly dedicated by the authors.

FOREWORD

POINTING THE WAY

DENNIS DeCONCINI
United States Senator from Arizona

Coming from Arizona, it's easy for me to relate to arthritis. Because our climate is stable and lots of people go there seeking relief, we have one of the highest per capita rates of the affliction in the United States. Rheumatoid arthritis is so cruel and its effects are so dramatic that even though I have known some arthritics who have had substantial recovery, I have always thought of it as a tragedy without relief.

When I came to Washington, I had no idea what our government was doing in this field, but I soon learned that it was substantial, and I became involved. Over the years, I have had progressively more influence on the allocation of federal moneys for arthritis research.

More recently, through a constituent named Barbara Matia, I heard about Dr. Thomas McPherson Brown. Four or five years ago she came to my office with a thick file about his work, and one day a few weeks later, while I was on a long flight, I took it out of my briefcase for what I thought would be a quick look. It was fascinating, and I didn't put it down until I had read it from beginning to end. Shortly after that, Barbara brought Dr. Brown to my office. He has pioneered in this field for a lifetime, and his evidence in support of the infectious view of arthritis is very convincing. I have become a believer.

I am a fiscal conservative, but I have always felt that medical research was the worst possible place to save money. Arthritis is the world's most widespread disease, and its cost in terms of suffering, lost productivity, and the expense of treatment is beyond calculating. It is the responsibility of government to invest in the kind of scientific query, especially in studying the infectious causes of arthritis, that will establish its ultimate cure. To that end, I have added to the 1988 Senate appropriations for Labor, Health & Human Resources & Education a $3-million item earmarked specifically for research into the infectious nature of the disease.

I believe the day will come when arthritis will not only be cured, but will be eliminated. We will all be in debt to Thomas McPherson Brown for pointing the way.

This book does not substitute for the medical advice and supervision of your personal physician. No medical therapy should be undertaken except under the direction of a physician.

The Road Back offers important new insights into the infectious nature of rheumatoid arthritis and provides detailed guidelines for antibiotic therapy. If it has been medically determined that you are suffering from a form of rheumatoid arthritis, we believe your physician would welcome the opportunity to read this book, to learn more about the infectious etiology of this disease and its safe, effective treatment.

Physicians who would like more information about seminars, tapes, and learning aids on the infectious etiology of rheumatoid arthritis or on its diagnosis and treatment are invited to write or call:

Office of Professional Education
Arthritis Institute
National Hospital for Orthopedics and Rehabilitation
2455 Army Navy Drive
Arlington, Virginia 22206
1-703-553-2431

Patients, physicians, and others wishing to receive periodic updates on research, treatment, legislation, and reimbursement policies related to rheumatoid arthritis should write:

National Arthritis Advocacy
Post Office Box 70438
Washington, D.C. 20024

CHAPTER 1

The Road Back

Arthritis has been with the human race longer than any other known disease—perhaps since our most distant ancestors first stood upright. But unlike other scourges of the ancient past, it is still very much with us: in addition to being man's oldest affliction, it is also the most widespread, affecting one out of every seven people on the planet.

It is not a minor disorder or a simple inconvenience. Arthritis can disfigure hands, twist spines, paralyze joints, weaken the connective tissue in hearts and other vital organs, and create fatigue, intense depression, and agonizing pain. Today, over a hundred different forms of the disease collectively afflict some 37 million Americans, and that number is growing at a rate of over a million cases every year. The price, including various forms of treatment and the cost of lost productivity, has been estimated at as much as $50 billion a year, or $1 billion a week, in this country alone.

The reason these numbers remain so astronomical even in this age of advanced technology is that pharmaceutical research took a serious wrong turn just before the middle of this century, one that created a forty-year detour in the search for the cause and cure of rheumatoid arthritis. As a result of that wrong turn, the American medical establishment was left with little choice but to treat the disease as an act of God. Patients were told they were born to have the disease through heredity, or that it was produced by stress, injury, a glandular defect, or aging, and that nothing could be done to avoid it or to cure it. For many years since that time, the approach to treatment has been purely symptomatic.

A *TRAGIC FAILURE*

Treatment of the symptoms of rheumatoid arthritis is now one of America's major industries. Judged purely in terms of profits, it is among the most successful. Judged by results, it is a tragic failure.

Even forty years ago, it was obvious that none of these speculations on the probable mechanism of rheumatoid arthritis held water. It is true that there are families in which arthritis is endemic, but there are many other instances in which there has been only a single case in three generations, which of course confutes the hereditary concept. As to aging as a cause, one only has to consider the hundreds of thousands of victims of juvenile rheumatoid arthritis or the millions of arthritics who are still in their teens and twenties. Stress is even less substantial: most highly stressed people never get arthritis, and many people who have very little stress in their lives suddenly find themselves afflicted. Another "explanation" for the disease is that it is caused or can be cured by diet. Nearly every disease is influenced to a certain extent by what we eat, and the nutritional link to arthritis has been worked over hundreds of different ways. There is some evidence, for example, that Eskimos have less arthritis than the rest of us—but there is no clear proof that it is because they consume so much fish oil.

The effect of all this confusion was a general abrogation of responsibility for finding the real cause of the disease, and pharmaceutical companies turned their attention elsewhere;

the formulation and manufacture of arthritis pain relievers eventually would become one of the biggest businesses in the world.

Cortisone came along at about that time, and its dramatic initial impact on the inflammation and pain of rheumatoid arthritis was interpreted at first as an indication that the basic cause of the disease was a glandular deficiency. Cortisone was a natural body product, after all, and if it worked so well on arthritis, it must be that the arthritic's body wasn't producing the required amount. From there it was a short step to characterizing arthritis as an autoimmune response. This view of the disease as the body fighting its own cells was a convenient one, and this convenience soon translated into unyielding dogma.

There were three basic problems with the autoimmune theory. It was accepted before it was proven. It went against prior evidence. It was based on flawed logic. A fourth problem was that it essentially derailed all further efforts to pursue an understanding of the real cause of the disease for the next three decades.

GOING FOR THE CAUSE

As a young clinician and researcher in this field, I was aware that no major disease had ever been understood or conquered until its cause had been identified. I also knew that serendipity favors medical research only when the investigator is on the right path to begin with, and that nobody ever stumbled onto the North Pole while they were headed south. The problem of finding the right starting place in the search for the cause of rheumatoid arthritis was comparable to coming from another culture and being asked to explain the exploded atomic bomb; no doubt one of the last things one would think of is the splitting of the atom. But I was determined to find the right starting point, the one that pointed due north to the cause.

The first clue I had that the cause of rheumatoid arthritis was an infectious agent that produced a damaging type of allergic reaction came from a simple clinical observation.

I was a third-year medical student at Johns Hopkins, using my free time to work in the Arthritis Clinic; it was an area in which the patients had great needs, and little was known. Gold salts were being administered, as they are today, and almost invariably the patient became much worse following the first injection. Yet with subsequent weekly injections, most patients gradually improved. This seemed to indicate that there was a hidden causative factor that was being stirred up at the start, but with continued treatment that factor was being reduced.

At the time the rest of the arthritis research establishment embarked on this long excursion down the byway of symptomatic treatment, I took on new duties as professor and chairman of the Department of Medicine at George Washington University in Washington, D.C. I was also a member of the American Rheumatism Association Committee on Public Relations, a body whose principal function was to interpret medical dogma for the American consumer. As director of the Department of Medicine, with philosophical as well as scientific responsibilities to the students, I soon found myself compelled to take a stand against the trend, by then widespread, toward the indiscriminate use of large doses of cortisone for pain relief in arthritis.

In large doses, cortisone weakens the immune system, and simple logic tells us this can only lead to trouble; the benefits of pain relief are soon offset by serious complications associated with the reduction of the body's natural defense mechanism. We had already seen tuberculosis become activated in the presence of cortisone treatment, as well as the transformation of chicken pox and measles from mild childhood illnesses into lethal disease processes due to uncontrolled pneumonia and meningitis that developed when the immunity was weakened.

Conversely, I wasn't against the use of cortisone altogether.

Small doses had been shown to help arthritics by modifying their allergic state, allowing other medicines to become more effective. But large doses had the opposite effect, interfering with any treatment program that depended on the immune system for its support.

THE FIRST VICTIM OF CORTISONE

Ironically, it was the advent of cortisone, which was an undeniably valuable discovery, that pulled the rug out from under any attempt to go for the cause of rheumatoid arthritis. The actual event when this occurred was a meeting of the American Rheumatism Association in Atlantic City in the early 1950s. I was one of five panelists invited to discuss cortisone and its use.

At that time, cortisone was still a very expensive drug to manufacture, and the head of the arthritis program at the National Institutes of Health, a Dr. Joseph Bunim, was advocating a cortisone subsidy from Congress. He was primarily a researcher rather than a practitioner, and he disregarded the risks in favor of the drug's dramatic effect on the relief of pain. Dr. Bunim declared, as did the drug's discoverer, that cortisone for arthritis was really comparable to insulin for diabetes, and that any difficulties with the drug could be overcome with further research.

The moderator opened the panel discussion before an audience of several thousand physicians by asking me for my views in regard to the use of cortisone. I took a deep breath and said that in large doses it was an extremely dangerous drug—that it should be used sparingly if at all. My statement was equivalent to coming out against mother's milk; I knew I was stepping into the fiery furnace, but I had no choice.

Dr. Bunim didn't take it at all well. He felt that winning a consensus of this audience of doctors was essential to gain final approval for the subsidy legislation then in Congress, and my remarks could do great harm to his efforts. He stood up and said in a voice shaking with fury that my statement was totally irresponsible.

The moderator, who was from the Mayo Clinic where cortisone had been initially developed, objected to Bunim's response. He said that I had a perfect right to my views, that the Association appreciated hearing them, and that Dr. Bunim's comments were uncalled for. As Bunim settled angrily into his seat, I could see my fortunes settling with him; I knew that from that time on I would be in trouble with the Establishment. Cortisone was indeed a lethal weapon, and one of its first victims was the voice of opposition.

A number of physicians in the audience came up to the stage after the meeting and congratulated me for taking a strong stand, saying that they, too, had encountered some serious problems with the drug. But within two weeks, I received a call from an officer of the American Rheumatism Association asking politely if I would be willing to withdraw from membership on the Public Relations committee. He told me he wanted to be sure that others in the membership would have the opportunity to serve in this responsible and highly visible position. I laughed and said, "Come on, George, who are you kidding? You guys are going to be sore at me forever."

I also told him that as chairman of the Department of Medicine, I said what I did because I had a responsibility to the truth. He said my remarks about cortisone had nothing to do with it. There was no doubt where all this was going, and I had neither the time nor the inclination to pursue a course that could only end in futility and rancor, so I withdrew my name.

Shortly afterward, Congress voted to subsidize the production of cortisone.

From that time on, our funding for research into the cause of arthritis at George Washington University nearly disappeared and we had to scrounge for every penny.

The main thrust of arthritis research in America spent itself unproductively in the cul-de-sac of metabolic dysfunction and autoimmunity for the next thirty years. It is only in the past decade that it began at last to find its way back to the main road.

RETURNING TO THE MAIN ROAD

When an inexperienced hunting dog is first exposed to game, he uses all of his energy searching for tracks in an open field, running in circles, chasing after every lead regardless of how fresh or stale. A researcher in the cause of arthritis is faced with the same apparently endless number of possibilities, with the potential for at least as much frustration and hopelessness. But like the hunting dog, he eventually learns which directions are most likely to be productive and he begins to establish a set of priorities. And he starts to get results.

This book describes how the dogs that have been hunting for the infectious cause of arthritis eventually got smart, what they found, and why they are now about to become the Most Popular Breed.

It deals with all the rheumatoid forms of arthritis, which means every form except osteoarthritis. With that single exception, all the many and varied types of this affliction have an inflammatory component, they all show evidence of connective-tissue damage, and they all are under the aegis of a process which resembles the autoimmune reaction.

A real autoimmune reaction is the body fighting its own cells. In rheumatoid arthritis, the body does not attack its own cells as the primary target. What is called the autoimmune reaction in all these forms of arthritis is actually the body's natural defense against an infection in the connective tissues. The body attacks disease agents that cling to the cells or are embedded within them. The infectious agent, and the body's reaction, cause the inflammation, the pain, and the eventual disfigurement of rheumatoid arthritis. When the body makes that response, it also attacks the cell to which the disease agent is connected. But if the agent is taken away, the body immediately stops the attack.

This process differs from true autoimmunity in that one important respect. It can be stopped, and true autoimmunity cannot.

This book is about how those inflammatory forms of arthritis begin, how they operate in the body, and how they can be treated successfully. The last pieces of one of the most complex puzzles in medicine are falling into place.

THE MYTH OF AUTOIMMUNITY

During the long detour, rheumatoid arthritis was treated with drugs that address its symptoms by changing the body's metabolism. The myth of autoimmunity has been used both as the justification for such a drastic approach and as the excuse for its inevitable failure. These drugs are extremely powerful and they will slow down the arthritic reaction, but often at a terrible price; they can damage the retina in the eyes, destroy the marrow in the bones, cause the kidneys to fail, and even kill the patient. One of them, gold, achieved the worst record for mortality of any prescription product on the market.

The reason the effects of metabolic drugs don't endure, so this circular logic goes, is that the autoimmune reaction is unstoppable. The real reason metabolic drugs don't hold up is that they merely mask the symptoms of the disease while they ignore its cause.

Because the prospects seemed so hopeless, doctors have been inclined to ignore the suggestive early symptoms and hope they will go away. Ask anyone you know who suffers from serious rheumatoid arthritis, and the chances are you will hear that it started as a lesser affliction.

Because the autoimmune theory has been taught in most medical schools for the past half-century, rheumatoid arthritis carries with it the stigma of a persistent, downhill condition that can never be cured. Doctors hate that kind of disease, and many of them will diagnose its onset as bursitis, lumbago, tendonitis, polymyositis, synovitis, or osteoarthritis so they can defer dealing with an unstoppable process. That way, a doctor can still do what seems to be best for the patient without having to bring in his heavy artillery such as gold, Plaquenil, chloroquine, penicillamine, Cytoxan, Imuran, or methotrexate to treat the early stages. He can gain a year or two by assuming it's something else.

A THERAPEUTIC PROBE

In their approach to many other diseases, doctors are able to complete a tentative diagnosis by what they call a therapeutic probe. This is the use of a medicine to see if it will relieve a condition—and if it does, the therapy helps verify what the patient is suffering from. But what responsible physician wants to risk inducing blindness or fatal kidney damage just to diagnose or relieve a little bursitis? The doctor has been as badly trapped by the autoimmune theory as his patients.

The infectious view of rheumatoid arthritis has been around far longer than the metabolic theory, but the infectious process is highly complicated, difficult to visualize, and until recently was extremely resistant to the traditional proofs of scientific research. Meanwhile, the metabolic bandwagon achieved such momentum during its forty-year roll, few doctors were aware of alternative treatments.

Today that is no longer the case. In some forms of rheumatoid arthritis the specific infectious agent, such as a mycoplasma or a spirochete, has already been identified. In others it is strongly suspected. There is always a gap in medicine between research results and their application, and most physicians have not yet been trained in dealing with arthritis as an infection—or, more precisely, an infectious allergy or hypersensitivity. But today, instead of prescribing a metabolic drug to suppress the symptoms, if the physician uses the right antibiotic as a therapeutic probe with the right frequency and dosage and with anti-inflammatory support, he can relieve the symptoms and confirm the diagnosis without placing the patient's life at risk.

And, at long last, he can begin to put the disease in remission and follow the clear, fresh tracks toward the ultimate cure.

CHAPTER 2

Myra Frank

Several years ago I received quite a number of patients from northwest Iowa. The word had gotten around that I had an approach to arthritis that could get results where others didn't, and Myra Frank came to me on such a referral.

Her father called me one morning and asked if I could help his daughter. He said she was twenty-one and desperately ill with rheumatoid arthritis. She had been to the Mayo Clinic where they put her on penicillamine, one of the relatively new drugs at that time; it had the risky component of producing suppression of the bone marrow in some people, and, unfortunately, she was one of the victims of that effect. When he called me, Myra had been sent home, but another hospital had found her white blood cell count was only 700, about 10 percent of what it should be to take care of infection. Ironically, the penicillamine had relieved none of her symptoms before going on to cause this toxic reaction.

I suggested that Mr. Frank take his daughter back to the Mayo Clinic, that they should take responsibility for her condition, but he said Myra refused to go back, that by that time she didn't like doctors at all, she didn't trust them and was thoroughly disillusioned. I made arrangements to get her admitted to the National Hospital at the earliest possible date.

When she arrived, it was obvious that she was every bit as sick as her father had said. She had large, draining abscesses scattered all over her body. Some of them were very deep and went down into the muscle layer. She was obviously frightened and had very little trust of any doctor, including myself. One of my major jobs, I saw at the outset, was to get her to accept some element of hope.

Little by little, we made progress in that direction. She already had been taken off the penicillamine, and the hospital at home had put her on high levels of cortisone in its place; we ended that as well, starting treatment with antibiotics and a low level of steroids to block some of the reaction. She began to pick up. And much to my amazement, her white cells actually began to come up as well.

Generally speaking, when a patient is suffering from aplastic anemia because drugs have stopped the bone marrow from forming cells, the blood levels never come back again and that's the end of it. But Myra's did. I never saw it happen before or since.

Gradually she improved in other ways as well. Eventually, she was healthy enough that one of the plastic surgeons at the hospital began a series of skin transplants to cover the large areas of her backside and leg that had become totally denuded of skin by her reaction to penicillamine.

Then we began to treat her arthritis, which was extremely severe. And that too began to improve.

At each slow step of the way, I could see that we were changing her attitude about medicine and about her disease. We were winning her respect. And most important of all, she was regaining her self-confidence.

Several years have passed. Myra still has active arthritis, but it is easily controlled now under the program. She has had some joint replacements. She has gotten to be strong. She drives a car. She travels around the world. And she has appeared more than once before committees of the Congress of the United States to tell the story of her treatment and recovery. She is an excellent example of someone who has been brought back from a condition that was truly hopeless.

HER STORY

When I was twelve years old, I lived with my parents and two sisters on our farm in Cherokee, Iowa. I was in the seventh grade and very athletic, probably more than even most of the boys in my class. I played every kind of game there was, and I was good at them all. At five feet seven inches and 130 pounds, I was also big for my age, and when we made up teams I was always the first kid my friends and classmates selected to be on their side. One day, a bump appeared on my elbow, and I went to the school nurse. She took one look and told me she thought it was rheumatoid arthritis. That's something old people get, I thought to myself, and I laughed. I had no idea that the childhood I had known was about to end.

The nurse told my parents that I should see our family doctor. When I did, he said the nurse was right about the bump, and he referred me to an arthritis specialist at the University of Iowa Hospital. So we drove six hours to Iowa City, the doctors there told me the same thing I had heard before, and then they sent me home. They didn't seem to be making a big deal out of it, and I didn't think it was a big deal either.

But they kept asking me to come back.

At first, because of my age, I went to pediatrics, but after a year or so they started sending me to rheumatology. By then, if I still had doubts about what lay ahead, all I had to do was look around at the other kids and older patients to get a preview of what was in store. They looked absolutely horrible, and I knew they were really suffering. It was scary, and I'd come out of there feeling very depressed.

My own condition began going downhill fast. My joints ached, and I lost most of my old energy. More subtly, the enthusiasm and hopefulness and excitement for the future that were always a part of my earlier life had drained out of me. I was still at the beginning, still a child, but within those first several months my horizons became shorter and shorter until I deliberately stopped thinking about the future at all. The hospital still hadn't started me on any medication stronger than aspirin, but by the end of the first year I was taking twenty pills a day and that still wasn't enough to do the job. My appetite had fallen off, I had lost twenty pounds, and big knobs started to appear on most of my joints. Because my knee joints began to deteriorate, at a time when my classmates were still growing, I began to get shorter. And I was in pain.

My friends treated me differently, probably because it was so scary for them to see this happening to someone they knew who had been so strong and athletic. In just a few months, I went from being the first one picked to being the last one anyone wanted on his or her team, and that hurt terribly. Pretty soon, I couldn't play at all. I would go to school, come home, and go to bed. I didn't talk to people about my illness. My mother sat down on the edge of my bed one afternoon and asked me to tell her how I felt—not just physically, but how I felt about what was happening to me. I told her I didn't want to talk about it. I wouldn't talk to anyone about it.

There's a lot of height in my family: my father is six feet seven inches, one sister is six feet, and the other sister is five feet ten inches. Both girls are younger than I, but they grew beyond me and eventually became basketball players in high school. I probably would have been tall too, but I stopped growing at the age of thirteen. I suspect the cortisone had something to do with it—my sisters both grew a couple of inches the last two years in high school.

The disease began to affect my marks in school. Through the seventh grade I had been pretty much a straight *A* student, but when I was a freshman in high school I got my first *D*. I just didn't have the concentration to study anymore.

During all of these changes, there was one constant: I kept getting in the family car every few months and riding the six hours each way to the hospital in Iowa City. Once I got there, the doctors would seat me on the examining table and shake their heads knowingly about how much worse I was getting, and often a whole team of young doctors or medical students would poke my joints and pull me this way and that. I soon grew to feel that I was making this long journey for the benefit of the doctors, to demonstrate how a disease operates and to reassure them that nature was running its proper course. Once in a while one of them would tell my parents that maybe we would get lucky and the disease would eventually "burn itself out," something that apparently can happen in very rare instances of the juvenile form of the disease. But the condition continued through my adolescence, and it was decided that I didn't have the juvenile form. Never once in the first three years did I hear anyone talk of doing a single thing to make me better.

That changed suddenly during my sophomore year of high school, as I entered the fourth year of the disease. By then I had a lot of joint damage, especially in my hands, and I was badly crippled. On one of my visits to Iowa City, the doctors told me they were going to put me on cortisone. Nobody suggested it would be a cure, but I was told it would help for a while with the symptoms.

The morning after the first treatment I felt so good I almost jumped out of bed. That's the way cortisone is at the beginning. And it wasn't just the first day: it worked well for the next couple of years, and got me back in the mainstream. I look back on cortisone as the reason I was able to get through high school. My grades came back up, and my spirits improved enormously.

I still look back on those high school years as including some very good times. I played drums in the marching band. I attended every athletic event there was, and even though I could no longer participate, I especially loved watching my sisters play basketball. I went to proms and homecoming dances and was in the National Honor Society. And through it all, even though I couldn't bring myself to talk with them about my arthritis, I knew I had a wonderful, loving family behind me.

But cortisone is one of those drugs you're not supposed to take in large quantities or for long periods, and so by the end of my senior year the doctors tried tapering me off. I could never stop cortisone altogether because by this time my body had stopped producing it naturally and I needed to keep up a small maintenance level just to stay alive.

They didn't taper me off in time. I began to develop side effects from the large earlier doses. Most particularly, I began to experience a breakdown of my skin tissue. Every time I banged against something or got a scratch or small puncture, I would develop sores and lesions. My arthritis came back at the same time, even worse than it had been before.

On the strength of my grades during the final three years of high school I enrolled at Iowa State University, but my condition was deteriorating fast. I got a bike so I could cover the sometimes long distances between classes, and I rode it through snow and in all kinds of weather. But I found that the energy I was using to get to class was all the energy I had, and there was nothing left for the work. I would have to sleep on campus a lot, and when I came home to my dorm I was so tired from the return trip that I couldn't study there either. At the end of my second year, I went home to Cherokee for the summer vacation and I got a letter from the school saying I had flunked out. I knew I had worked as hard as I was able, and it was a terrible blow.

Once the doctors had reduced my cortisone, they decided to try injecting me with gold. I can't remember now what the treatments cost, but they were terribly expensive. One of the side effects of gold can be kidney failure, and a first indicator that the gold is attacking the kidneys is protein in the urine. The protein showed up in tests after just a few months, and so the gold was stopped. It hadn't seemed to do a thing to improve my arthritis, and when they stopped giving it to me I didn't feel any different either.

The doctors switched to Plaquenil, which had been developed initially to fight malaria. Although I developed no side effects, I also showed no signs that it was doing my arthritis any good, so after six months they stopped that treatment as well and switched back to gold. All together, I was on the gold for about a year, until they had to stop it permanently.

By this time I was feeling very sick. I had no energy, was seriously anemic, in a lot of pain, and very depressed. I also had the feeling that I should be trying harder, but I just didn't have the energy to do more than I did. And I didn't like my family and friends to have to see what I was going through, so I made an effort to pretend that everything was fine. That strategy didn't fool anyone around me—it was perfectly obvious that I was in terrible shape—but because I spent so much time pretending, I never was able to come to terms with what was really happening to me.

I did have some good friends who stuck by me, and I often wondered what they were thinking—about me, about my disease, and about how I was handling myself. In a way, thinking about their reactions was as close as I dared get to thinking about where my life was going.

When I had left college I was majoring in accounting, so I enrolled in a small technical school in Sheldon, about fifty miles from home, and tried to resume my studies. But it didn't work. It seemed as though trying to lead a normal, productive life only made the arthritis worse, and the more I ignored it, the more it demanded my attention. The problem wasn't just the arthritis; the side effects were getting more serious at the same time.

I began to lose skin. A large sore appeared on my rear, and new sores emerged on my fingers, all exuding pus and causing a lot of discomfort. My white blood cell count dropped steeply, so my body's ability to heal itself and its natural defense against infections were very weak. All these problems were explained as the natural side effects of cortisone and the other drugs I'd been given, and the doctors kept saying they wanted me to get off the cortisone—but they didn't know how to do it.

We decided it was time to try something different, so I left the university hospital in Iowa City and started seeing a doctor in Omaha, Nebraska. My dad was usually the one to make those decisions; I really didn't care one way or another. I didn't have a whole lot of hope that anyone was ever going to find any way to help me, and I guess I was getting pretty dejected about going back to places where we spent a lot of money and no one could tell us anything.

Even so, I still wasn't totally cynical about the doctors who had been treating me. During the whole course of the disease, a lot of people would approach me or my family and ask if we had tried carrot juice or cod liver oil or whatever the latest fad was, and we'd see stories in the newspapers at the supermarket checkouts about exotic cures of one kind or another, but we just ignored them all. I continued to believe that the doctors who had studied the disease would know about every treatment on the market, and that if they didn't tell me about it, it was because it didn't work.

I had an appointment to see the doctor in Omaha one Monday morning, so I came home from school in Sheldon the Friday before in order to spend the weekend with my family in Cherokee. It had been normal for me to run a fever of 100 or 101 over the previous year, and my weight had dropped to just around a hundred pounds. My dress was a size 5. I felt sick most of the time. That Sunday night, as we were all sitting at the dining room table after dinner, for no apparent reason and without any warning, I suddenly vomited. It happened again a short time later in the kitchen.

In addition to being slightly embarrassed, I felt even worse than usual. We knew I was going to see the doctor the next day, so after a while I sat in an easy chair beside the telephone, trying to get my mind off the way I felt by studying. My father recalls that a short time later he was reading in the living room, and when he heard me talking in the dining room, he assumed I was using the phone. Then he realized that I was mumbling incoherently, and when he came out to the dining room he found me bent over the side of the chair in convulsions. I don't remember anything until I woke up in the emergency room of our local hospital. They stopped the convulsions and put me in an ambulance to Omaha.

The doctors in Omaha stayed up with me all night, running tests, trying to find out what had happened. What they finally determined was that an infection from all the sores on my body had suddenly "turned on," and that my temperature had shot up to 105 as my system tried to fight it, producing the convulsions.

They gave me antibiotics to fight the infection. They also decided I needed to put on weight and they put me on a 4,000-calorie diet. I didn't gain any weight to speak of, and although the infection seemed to eventually diminish, the doctors were unable to heal the lesions. After a month in the hospital they sent me home, still covered with sores.

I went back to the technical college, but I knew by then that my further education was a lost cause and that I was going to have to stay close to home, because I couldn't take care of myself. Shortly afterward I saw an ad for a bookkeeper in Cherokee, and I resigned from the school and moved back in with my family.

During the following year, the side effects were always with me, and even though I managed to work fairly steadily on the new job, I had the feeling that I was sitting on a deadly bomb and that it was just about to explode. I had sores on the bottoms of my feet, and at the end of that year one of my feet suddenly began to swell. I knew that once more, the bomb was going off.

It was the weekend of a family reunion, and I just wasn't up to attending, so I stayed at home in bed. Dad must have been doing a lot of thinking about it, because when everyone came back, he walked into my bedroom and said, "What do you think about going up to Rochester, Minnesota, to the Mayo Clinic?"

I could feel the tears coming into my eyes. I was so sick of those places I never wanted to see another one. Each new hospital was a little farther away than the last, and I knew that none of them could do anything for me. I told him I was sure the Mayo Clinic would be just one more place where I was a guinea pig for the doctors to poke and probe, and that I'd get nothing out of it.

But as usual I said yes.

The doctors up at Mayo examined me thoroughly, and then told me it was time to try something a little different. They had a new drug called penicillamine.

I recognized the name. It was all the rage at the time; I had seen an article about it in the *National Enquirer* and knew that penicillamine had gone through the FDA double-blind study and showed great promise. But I also knew that cortisone and gold and Plaquenil and untold numbers of other "wonder drugs" had similarly gone through the double-blind tests with flying colors in their times, only to eventually fail badly in sustained clinical use. I agreed without much enthusiasm or hope, and the Mayo Clinic began yet another course of treatment.

While I was in Rochester, right at the beginning of the penicillamine therapy, a new sore erupted on my leg. It was only about the size of a quarter at the beginning, but it was really deep and was extremely painful. Meanwhile, the doctors at Mayo examined the sore on my rear that had been open for the past two years and decided to do a skin graft. The skin was so unhealthy that the graft failed. And the sore on my leg got deeper and more painful.

My white blood count was very low when I arrived in Rochester, and I was kept in isolation for the entire duration of my stay. Rochester was a long way for anyone to travel from Cherokee—about seven hours by car—and so my family only got up there a few times during the first month, and I had one or two visits from a girlfriend I'd known since high school who had stuck with me through everything. One day the doctor came in and told me that I could expect to be in there for another three or four months. When he left I cried and cried, and no matter how much I wanted to stop I couldn't turn off the tears.

I had plenty of time to think while I lay there in isolation; I wasn't allowed to get out of bed even to go to the bathroom. I didn't like the way my life was going. I couldn't even bring myself to consider the future, but I knew in the back of my mind that the day was going to come soon when I would be truly helpless, and I would be dependent on someone else to take care of me. If I had any doubts, they were dispelled one day when a hospital social worker or psychologist came into my room and started to counsel me on how to accept my disease. She told me I could expect to be in a wheelchair in the not-too-distant future. I think she was feeling me out to determine how realistic I was about what lay ahead.

My father was visiting with me at the time she appeared, and I noticed during her little talk that he turned white as a sheet. Perhaps her remarks had been for his benefit as well, because certainly what she was telling me would have an impact on the whole family. As for me, instead of being shocking, the revelation was a matter of real indifference; I didn't think of myself as being a part of life at that point anyway, and I listened to her with no particular reaction. When she left the room, I realized with some surprise that my father was furious. "Don't listen to a word she said," he told me. "She doesn't know what she's talking about."

Soon after that, my father decided on another, completely different course of action. He came up one weekend in the middle of my second month and told me about a story he had seen in an Iowa newspaper, during the same family reunion when he had heard about the Mayo Clinic. The article was about a rheumatoid arthritic named Don Knop, a young college student from Iowa who had gone to the National Hospital outside Washington and been treated by a doctor named Thomas McPherson Brown. It said Knop's arthritis was now under control, that he was able to function normally with no exotic chemicals and no side effects. When my father showed me the clipping, I read it quickly and let it drop on the bed, then turned my face away and stared out the window at the construction going on outside in a world I didn't seem to be a part of. I was certain this was just one more beginning of another painful and inevitable defeat. It was more than I could bear.

My father patiently explained that he had learned far more about the story than was in the newspaper. He said he had met the Knop family and had heard of their son's experience at first hand. He had even listened to a tape recording that Dr. Brown had given them on the nature of their son's disease, its prognosis under the treatment he had begun, and the course it would follow to its conclusion.

"Conclusion" was a word I had never heard before in the whole decade of my ordeal. It didn't inspire the least bit of hope, but I realized when my father said it that no one ever before had talked about the possibility of my disease coming to an end. Dad went on and on; he was filled with excitement, and he was trying to pass some of it to me.

But instead of the reaction he was looking for, all he got from me was tears. He asked if I could explain why I was crying, and all I could say, over and over, was, "I don't know. I don't know."

But looking back on it, I think I do. I usually cried only when I was facing a new treatment or hospital. Maybe it forced me to think of the future. After ten years of torture and heartbreak, I had become terrified of hope; I knew where it would lead. I couldn't bear to consider the possibility that he might be right.

Two things happened during that visit. My father finally got me to agree to go to Washington to meet Dr. Brown, with whom he had already made an appointment. And, because the doctors apparently couldn't think of anything else to do with me, I was told to "go home and wait it out"; so I left the Mayo Clinic.

Because I was still continuing the penicillamine therapy, arrangements were made for me to have my blood and urine tested every two weeks at our local hospital for toxicity.

The trip to Washington was scheduled for about ninety days after my release from Mayo, on the twelfth of December. About a month before that date, I went into our hospital for the regular biweekly tests, and when I returned home I felt really sick. There was nothing alarming in this, because I felt sick almost all the time. I went to my room and lay down on the bed. I hadn't been lying there for more than a few minutes when the phone rang; it was the doctor who monitored the tests, telling my mother she had to get me back to the hospital as soon as possible. My white count had dropped to 700, which is very, very bad. In fact, they were afraid they might not be able to get it back up again.

My parents remember the times they visited me during the next couple of days while I was in isolation; my skin was gray, and they were frightened that I wasn't going to make it. The simple act of turning slightly in the bed produced pure agony. For the first time, I sensed the possibility that I might be about to die.

The local doctor ended the penicillamine therapy immediately, then raised my cortisone to an extremely high level; a little later my white count began to rise in response. The crisis passed. I stayed off the penicillamine, which should never have been prescribed for me in the first place with my low white count, and a month later I went to Washington.

I met Dr. Brown. We talked for a long time, and he explained to me how arthritis occurs; it was the first time anyone had discussed my illness with me in terms of its cause. He then explained what he was going to do to help me, and why simple antibiotic therapy would work. That was another first; no one else had discussed results, because in no previous treatment had positive results been a realistic possibility. At the end of that first meeting I was finally able to look at the future for the first time in ten years, not as something to be feared, but with hope.

I stayed at the hospital for less than a month, and by the time I went home I could already feel the difference. I had more energy. I was no longer smothered by depression. I felt better. My lesions and sores closed and began at last to heal. I had some skin grafts, and this time they worked. A few months later, I felt well enough to return to school—not at the technical college near my home, but back at Iowa State.

I graduated in 1983 with a degree in accounting. That September I got a job as an auditor with the Army Audit Agency, an opening I heard about from someone I met at the National Hospital, and I just recently moved to a similar job with the Office of the Inspector General. In just those few months, the world opened up to me again and I walked back into it.

I wrote to most of the doctors who had treated me since I was a child and told them about the astonishing thing that had finally happened. I gave them all the information about the causes and mechanism of arthritis that I had learned from Dr. Brown and from scientific papers that he and other researchers have published in medical journals. I described the treatment and my recovery. I felt my greatest responsibility now was to pass along the secret of new life for use on other patients they might treat for the same disease.

Several doctors wrote back. A rheumatologist from the Mayo Clinic told me that this kind of thing happens now and then in rheumatoid arthritis, and that nobody really knows why—it's just a matter of timing. He suggested that my treatment in Washington probably had nothing to do with my getting well. A doctor in Iowa City told me there was no scientific proof for the treatment I had received at the Arthritis Institute, and he said that such proof could only be derived from six-month double-blind studies—the same studies through which the drugs that nearly killed me had all passed with flying colors before displaying any of their lethal effects. Both letters made me very angry.

The doctor from Omaha was an internist, not a rheumatologist, and he wrote back too. He said he had heard of Dr. Brown and was very interested in how things were going; he asked me to keep him posted. Unlike the other two doctors, he wasn't defending an entrenched position, and he was willing to listen to his patient. I felt he really cared.

I remember a few of the other things I heard about rheumatoid arthritis from the Mayo Clinic and from a lot of other doctors and hospitals, and I have the choice of believing those things or believing my own experience. And I'm not alone; I met and talked with many other patients whose arthritis has been brought under control or into complete remission by Dr. Brown's treatment—there are over ten thousand of them. Today I don't sit in a wheelchair, and I don't expect I ever will. Instead, I have a wonderful, productive career and travel all over the world.

I have a life.

At last.

CHAPTER 3

The Golden Calf and Other Stories

Most physicians who treat arthritis tell their patients that there is a certain amount of risk in whatever medication they prescribe, but that there is a bigger risk in the disease. There are two important things, however, that most doctors *don't* tell their patients about that same medication.

They don't tell them that it will end up curing the disease or stopping its progress. Because it won't.

They don't tell them that the medication will eventually wear out, that it will stop working. But it will.

If the patient is incurring a serious risk by taking a drug that will wear out, that is a very different thing from taking the same risk with a medicine that will keep on working or that offers an outside chance of sustaining control. None of the traditional drugs prescribed for rheumatoid arthritis has an outside chance of sustaining control, and not one has ever cured a single case. All drugs that have been created specifically for treating arthritis eventually lose their effectiveness. That's why there are so many of them: the drug companies have to keep on bringing out something new to replace the previous drugs as they give out.

In the late 1970s, at the World Congress of Rheumatology in San Francisco, I gave a paper suggesting the joint scan as a means of determining whether the various forms of medication were helping to improve patient health; it was the first proposal for an objective measure of drug efficacy. Coincidentally, at the very same time that paper was presented, penicillamine was announced as the new drug that would cure arthritis. Penicillamine had been a big hit in England, and it got a lot of attention in the American press as a result. And no one paid the slightest attention to the proposal that we establish a scientific means for determining whether these drugs were really doing all the things that were being claimed for them.

Of course, the other thing our paper showed was that tetracycline did indeed produce improvements that were measurable in the joint scans, and that those improvements endured.

Two years later, the discovery was made that penicillamine produced aplastic anemia, and its luster began to diminish. In fact, by the time penicillamine was introduced in the United States, the medical community in England was already becoming aware that there could be some slight problems with it—that its benefits didn't last, and that its other effects were potentially lethal. But while they were waking up to these horrors on one side of the Atlantic, the medical world was celebrating this same product as the new Silver Bullet on the other.

SLIPPING BY THE DOUBLE-BLIND

Most of the troubles with these wonder cures appear late, usually just past the six-month double-blind testing period. As a result, the screening agencies that are supposed to be watching these things have left the job, and nobody monitors the changes that are taking place. The literature is already out, and it gives the impression of a sustained improvement because the drug worked for the first six months and everyone assumes that the trend will continue on the same upward curve. In reality, what happens instead is that the curve almost inevitably goes down.

With tetracycline, on the other hand, I have not seen any toxic effects in forty years in anybody. The drug is used in low doses, widely spaced to avoid sensitization; the higher the physician has to go in dosage, the wider the spaces. Extreme cases can be treated intravenously, which avoids potential allergic responses by going into a part of the body where allergies don't take place. Tetracycline doesn't attack the part of germs where immunity is formed, so it can be used virtually forever without giving rise to immune strains of the organism it is fighting.

Because of these features, I have been able to treat patients from Washington or Texas or California or Alaska or Cairo, get them started on tetracycline therapy, and then send them back home to continue a program of no-risk recovery. All they need is some help from their family doctor, and it has been my experience that in most cases such doctors are very glad to learn of the technique and see it through to a successful conclusion. If there are any problems with a tetracycline patient going out of balance and his dosage needing to be changed, the doctor can call me back or make the adjustment on his own, but there is never any risk whatever of a toxic effect. Indeed, a lot of physicians continue to use the same technique on other sufferers from rheumatoid arthritis, so the benefits spread.

By comparison, it would be extremely questionable practice for a physician who was treating someone with gold or methotrexate, for example, to let the patient out of his sight for any longer than a few days, such as for a trip abroad or even a short vacation in another state. Things happen too quickly with that kind of medication. With gold, the main risks are damage to the kidneys and bone marrow and destruction of the process by which the body creates platelets. In Germany, the use of oral gold in the treatment of arthritis has been identified as the cause of platelet depression in two cases where the patient subsequently bled to death from a simple bruise.

Methotrexate is an anticancer drug that was designed to interfere with the immune system. Like cortisone, it produces its effect by blocking the antigen-antibody reaction, but also like cortisone it leaves the antigen ready to react again. It is an extremely toxic compound which can damage the liver and the lungs, and sooner or later the physician has to stop giving it. Meanwhile, the patient has started on a journey similar to the one on which Moses led the Israelites through the Red Sea. The waters part for a time, but the path is inevitably downward and the risk of drowning from the walls of water on either side increases with each successive step. No physician who has entered this course has ever proven to be as wise or as successful as Moses; no one has gotten a single patient across to the Promised Land.

RISKS VS. BENEFITS

This type of medicine gains its advantage through a much larger disadvantage, and its risks are immense. The advantage is short-term pain relief. The disadvantages are severe whiplash as the arthritis mechanism gathers new fury once the treatment is stopped, along with the strong possibility of destruction of the lungs, and of liver damage that can lead to uremia and death. (A 1987 study of the efficacy and safety of methotrexate therapy in rheumatoid arthritis at McMaster University in Ontario by Tugwell, Bennett, and Gent cites nausea, vomiting, anorexia, and diarrhea in 10 percent of the subjects surveyed, stomatitis in 6 percent, leukopenia, anemia, or thrombocytopenia in 3 percent, and "rare" instances of toxicity of the liver, kidneys, or lungs, possible malignancy, oligospermia, fever, gynecomastia, localized osteoporosis, and leukocytonbastic vasculitis. Therapy had to be discontinued in one-third of those surveyed because of these and other effects. Their conclusion? "If approved [by the FDA], the drug should be given to patients with rheumatoid arthritis refractory to first- and second-line agents, such as injectable gold and penicillamine, who provide informed consent.")

HANDICAPPING THE DOCTOR

The liabilities of these products place an enormous burden on the rheumatologists who use them, a burden which shifts the attention of the physician away from the disease and focuses it instead on monitoring the high-risk treatment. With those drugs that impair platelet formation, that monitoring can take the form of periodic checks of the bone marrow, a process which is not only very costly but extremely painful. And of course it keeps the patient on a very short tether.

A method of treatment which does not entail those liabilities of great risk, pain, expense, and inconvenience, on the other hand, frees both the doctor and the patient from the need for close monitoring. A general physician doesn't have the time to follow his patient as closely as a rheumatologist, but with tetracycline he doesn't have to. When I order a blood test for a patient on a program of antibiotic therapy, it isn't to see whether the patient is surviving the medication, but rather to measure factors such as sedimentation rate or hemoglobin level to determine our progress in combating the disease of arthritis.

Once more, the only treatment that has any hope of curing rheumatoid arthritis is one that addresses the cause. Treatments that deal with the problem by placing the symptoms in a state of suspension are doomed to fail over the long term, and often at a terrible price. Antibiotic therapy is the only approach that dries up the source. It may require great persistence on the part of both the doctor and the patient, but I don't believe there is any possible shortcut, now or in the future.

The number of arthritics in the population mounts each

year. Just a couple of years ago it was 34 million, and now it has risen to 37 million. About half those people suffer from straight rheumatoid arthritis, and if you add in the patients who are afflicted with a combination of rheumatoid and osteoarthritis, the number is at least 25 million.

OSTEOARTHRITIS IS DIFFERENT

Osteoarthritis is a noninflammatory form of arthritis that is hereditary and is considered to be incurable. It is characterized by calcium deposits which can accumulate on pressure points and impinge on nerves, so there is some pain associated with it, although it is different from the pain that goes with the rheumatoid form. I have found that as a rule, when an osteoarthritis patient complains bitterly about the disease, it is because there is a component of rheumatoid arthritis mixed in with it. Until fairly recently it was very difficult to demonstrate the presence of rheumatoid arthritis in that kind of combination, because the osteo obscured the picture. However, the bone and joint scan has greatly illuminated the picture in recent times by revealing inflammatory reactions associated with the calcium pressure points.

This population of perhaps 10 million arthritics who have both forms represents a major added challenge, because a safe method of treatment is needed to allow the physician to probe therapeutically. It makes no sense to probe a possible combination of osteo and rheumatoid with gold or penicillamine or Plaquenil because the drugs are so dangerous to begin with. Until the bone scanner came along, many physicians chose to deal with the problem by concluding it wasn't there: they said that there was no such combination, and that a patient had either osteo or rheumatoid but never both. We have found through our own use of the bone scanner and tests for the mycoplasma antibody that approximately half the cases of osteoarthritis involve some degree of the rheumatoid form.

TOWARD PREVENTION

One of the great advantages of the tetracycline approach is that it allows the use of a safe therapeutic probe early in the disease when the risks from many of the standard drugs outweigh their possible usefulness. Early treatment is far more effective than late management. The antibiotic approach has already opened the way for treatment to prevent arthritis.

CHAPTER 4

Lauriane Riley

(As told by her mother)

About a year ago, when Lauriane was two years old, she developed a fever and a rash. The fever came and went intermittently for about fourteen days, and she was tired a lot and lost her appetite, so we finally put her into the local hospital. Some tests were done, and the doctor told us she was suffering from juvenile rheumatoid arthritis.

Our first question was how serious was it, and the doctors said they didn't know, that we'd have to wait and see. It was a frustrating time. They prepared us for the worst, telling us that this was a crippling disease, but they couldn't really tell us anything tangible about *how* crippling, or how soon it would happen, and they sent her home after four days.

Lauriane had a little stiffness in her knees, and the doctors told us to watch them for swelling and unusual warmth. They prescribed aspirin, but the dosage soon proved too much for her stomach so we had to cut way back.

In the meantime, I spoke with a friend, Dr. Cecil Jacobson, and he told me about Dr. Brown at the Arthritis Institute. He encouraged me to get a second opinion, and if it agreed with the first to take Lauriane to the Arthritis Institute.

For the second opinion we went to a large hospital in Washington. They confirmed the original diagnosis and were even more pessimistic about what we could expect for Lauriane's future. While we were at the second hospital, I mentioned to the doctors there that we were considering taking her to Dr. Brown. They said they had heard of him, but they didn't say anything else, good or bad. I have a lot of respect for Dr. Jacobson, who is a well-known geneticist, and even though he does not specialize in arthritis I trusted his referral, so I didn't press the Washington doctors to say anything more.

Lauriane and I met with Dr. Brown two days later at the National Hospital. By that time her legs had started to become stiff, she was reluctant to walk, her sedimentation rate was abnormally high, and she was suffering from anemia. Dr. Brown treated her with small doses of oral antibiotic and within three weeks all of those symptoms had disappeared. Six months later, in a complete laboratory workup at the National Hospital, not a single sign of arthritis remained.

A year has passed since Dr. Brown treated Lauriane. She has not had a fever since he started the medication, and there is no trace of stiffness in her legs or any reluctance to do all of the normal things—running, playing—that healthy children do. She eats well, has grown normally, and has lots of energy. She is completely recovered.

CHAPTER 5

The Case for Early Detection and Treatment

When an earthquake is about to take place, something happens in nature that prefigures the coming cataclysm. Dogs howl, cats climb trees, and birds stop singing. Whatever it is that signals these other members of the animal kingdom, man alone remains oblivious to the warning, either because he can't detect it, or because he doesn't recognize its meaning. Nature provides similar advance notice of the advent of diseases. Over the years, it has become clear that there is a forerunner to the development of acute rheumatoid arthritis, and in taking histories and treating patients, I have learned to become suspicious when certain symptoms are mentioned.

FATIGUE: THE EARLY WARNING

The most important of all antecedents to the rheumatoid explosion, the first development symptom on which one can most reliably base the suspicion that rheumatoid arthritis is about to happen, is unexplained fatigue; it precedes almost every case I have ever treated, sometimes coming on a year before there is any particular discomfort in the joints.

The fatigue will be serious enough that the patient goes to the doctor, but the doctor doesn't know what he is looking for and as a rule he doesn't find anything. He tells the patient that he or she is working too hard or is under too much stress. Another gambit is to ask the patient's age, and then to suggest that when one gets to that point in life—whatever point it happens to be—one naturally slows down a bit. That way, the doctor can sound profound at the same time as he admits his ignorance, which is precisely the posture favored by most physicians when they haven't the foggiest idea what's happening.

The patient starts to become anxious; feeling tired and poorly is bad enough, but not knowing why is worse. Perhaps there is something else going on. Or perhaps, as the doctor seems to suggest, the patient expects too much from life or is not altogether balanced psychologically. People who are tired are also down emotionally, so these suggestions fall on fertile soil.

ANEMIA AND OTHER SIGNS

Sometimes the fatigue is accompanied by anemia, and the physician usually jumps at the chance to connect the two as effect and cause. And when he finds that the anemia doesn't respond to iron or vitamin B-12 or folic acid or liver or to any of the things that ordinarily tend to raise the blood count, the common stratagem is to blame the intransigence of the anemia on the patient's peculiar nature, which, in turn, adds to the patient's anxiety. Stress has been clearly identified as an accelerator of the disease process, so by now the doctor has become a part of the problem.

When the next symptom emerges, it is usually a troublesome joint. The common reaction at this point is for the doctor to diagnose it as a sprain, and when the patient can't recall any event that might explain such a result, the doctor blames it on the patient's faulty memory. The diagnosis seems to be vindicated when the joint pain subsides and disappears, as usually happens with these first small warning shots before the arthritis explodes.

We have found that when a patient first complains of fatigue, especially if there is any connection with joint complaints, a test of blood for mycoplasma antibodies will produce positive results. Moreover, many patients will display these results for mycoplasma antibodies when nothing else shows. I have reached the conclusion, through long experience in following thousands of such patients, that even in the absence of any other indicator, signs of mycoplasmas in the blood are a guarantee that the patient is eventually going to develop either rheumatoid arthritis or some other disease of the connective tissue unless treatment is started. And I have learned not to wait.

THE IMPORTANCE OF HISTORY

At this stage it is also possible to gain supporting evidence by going back into the patient's history. Many have had periods of fatigue before, and some can recall times when they were also suffering from depression, although most people have never spoken of the depression to anyone or looked at it from the viewpoint that it might be a symptom of something else. There is a certain amount of risk in admitting to either fatigue or depression, and most people would rather accept these symptoms as normal parts of growing up than take that risk in bringing them out for examination. I suspect that in most such cases, the fatigue and depression go back to early childhood.

Of course there are other disorders that can explain fatigue—such as mononucleosis, infectious hepatitis, or low thyroid function—and these should be on the physician's list of things to eliminate. But once they have been ruled out, the doctor should be suspicious of early rheumatoid disease, and not write it off as an emotional imbalance. This is particularly important because at the time the fatigue develops, the patient is also usually more tense and nervous. These traits may owe to natural worry about a symptom that cannot be explained, or they may be symptoms in themselves, as we know them to be at later stages of rheumatoid disease.

Many other psychological factors can appear in this early syndrome of arthritis: irritability, reduced mental acuity, slower motor skills, shorter attention span, hesitancy, and loss of confidence. These can be bothersome to anybody, but they are particularly frightening to older people, who often interpret them as early signs of senility or Alzheimer's disease.

Some pre-arthritics are extraordinarily sensitive to cold. I had one patient arrive in my office wearing a fur coat on a hot summer day. Others can be overly sensitive to heat. An impaired thermostat in either direction is a warning sign.

THE ATTACK

When the actual rheumatoid aspect finally shows itself, it is most commonly first seen in the small joints of the hands, feet, and ankles, although not always by any means. Regardless of where it begins, the real key to early rheumatoid disease is its migratory nature; it is an elusive Gypsy. Many people are misled by that nomadic feature into the belief that once it has left a particular area, it has cleared up. But it always comes back, becoming progressively more constant and more fixed.

From a treatment point of view, once the disease starts becoming localized, it is getting more serious. The migratory phase, before the body has started to encase the infectious agent inside its defensive walls of scars and inflammation, is considerably simpler to get at.

That is pretty much the way rheumatoid arthritis starts. In some cases it can tarry at one or another of these stages for months or even a few years, slight, insidious, mistaken for something else, often simply tolerated and ignored. In other cases it can explode overnight with a violence that leaves its victim suffering agonies in every joint.

It is interesting that people who experience an explosive onset often go into remission for a couple of years. Their immune systems have been shaken up to fight back hard, and protect them for a period following the attack. This action and reaction portrays a typical infectious process, and even when the arthritis finally returns after that kind of a start, it is frequently more responsive to treatment than the kind that seems to creep into the system a little bit at a time.

Viral pneumonia is a good prototype for what happens when a mycoplasma infection becomes fixed around a certain area. In the lung, the disease produces sections of what look like nodules of granulation material, inflamed tissues that are apparently fixed around the infectious organism and remain in position for months, producing the characteristic cough of the disease. I visualize the same thing happening in the joints, although it's a lot harder to see there; we seldom biopsy joint tissue, although doctors used to, because we have found that rheumatoid arthritis tends to produce excessive scars where the mycoplasmas cluster, and the biopsy produces more pain than the information is worth.

LETTING THE BODY DEFEND ITSELF

The physician has to pay careful attention to the body's defense mechanism as one of the primary aspects of the treatment of rheumatoid arthritis. He has to let the body do as much as it can to suppress the agents that cause the arthritis. That means carefully reducing the barriers which the body erects around the mycoplasmas so that they can be effectively purged without stimulating the production of the toxins that characterize the allergic flareup.

The doctor starts this process on first seeing the patient by giving some simple anti-inflammatory remedy such as aspirin, Bufferin, Ecotrin, or the like, the choice depending on how the patient's stomach responds; this assumes the disease is a fresh, new case and not severe. (I must admit that only about 5 percent of the patients in my own practice are in this category; as a rule, by the time a patient gets as far as the Arthritis Institute, the disease is pretty well advanced.) The purpose in using these mild anti-inflammatories is not to treat symptoms, but rather to permit the body to get through its own barriers. If the aspirin doesn't do the job, the doctor goes on to the encids: Clinoril, Naprosyn, Meclomen, Tolectin, Nalfon, Motrin, or similar drugs.

The doctor has to be continuously mindful of the mechanism, and not the symptoms, when he is treating the disease. This calls for a clear understanding of a very complex process (described in detail in Chapter 18) and a certain degree of tough-mindedness. The physician's main responsibility is to relieve the disease, not just to make the patient feel better without regard for what happens next.

CHAPTER 6

Talmadge Williams, Ph.D.

My problem started back in the middle seventies. I was working for a computer firm, and when I went for my annual physical checkup the doctor told me that the blood test had revealed traces of rheumatoid arthritis. I hadn't noticed any symptoms that would have made me suspect there was anything seriously wrong; in fact, the only unusual thing I could recall was minor—a slight tingling or numbness occasionally at the ends of my fingers—but no pain and no stiffness. The doctor took the blood test seriously, however, and sent me over to George Washington University Hospital.

The tests were repeated at the hospital, the new doctor confirmed the signs of arthritis, and I was given some pills and sent home. The pills were Naprosyn, an anti-inflammatory analgesic, which I was to take just a couple of times a week. I followed the hospital's directions for the next couple of years, and everything seemed to be fine.

One night I was sitting at my desk at home, studying for my work; I had to concentrate hard on learning about changes in my field of employment, which seemed to occur almost daily. Moreover, I was under a lot of family stress at the time. As I idly scratched my head during the study session that particular evening, I felt something sticky and, when I withdrew my hand, discovered blood on my fingers. In looking at the mirror a moment later, I saw that I had scratched a small hole in my scalp. I was annoyed with myself, but not at all alarmed. I interpreted the event as an indicator of the stress I was under, and nothing more.

After a few days, the hair around the lesion still had not started to grow back and I became concerned. I made an appointment with a dermatologist at Howard University Hospital and was given some salve, Lindex ointment, to help restore the hair. The doctor didn't exaggerate the problem of a small, self-inflicted scratch on my head, but he was more concerned with why it had happened so easily and why the hair had not come back on its own. He asked me about my medical history, and I told him about the rheumatoid arthritis. As soon as he heard that, he sent me over to see their rheumatologist.

The rheumatologist did some more tests, and the next day he called me and said, "Williams, you have lupus." He had me come back in, prescribed some medication, and the next day I was extremely sick. I decided it was time for me to head back to George Washington Hospital to talk with the doctor who had diagnosed my arthritis two years earlier.

Back at GW, my original doctor ran the standard tests again and told me I did not have lupus, but that my skin problem was related to the arthritis and it was time to change my treatment. He increased the amount of Naprosyn to twice the dosage, now taken three times every day. The condition quickly began to get worse. I saw swelling in my ankles and wrists, nodules came up on my elbow and wrist, and I started to become very stiff. He saw that the original medicine wasn't doing the job, so he decided to put me on gold.

The gold treatment consisted of fifty milligrams injected in my muscles every week. Each time I went over for the shot, they gave me blood and urine tests beforehand to make sure I wasn't having a reaction. The treatment was very costly—something in the neighborhood of $140 every week, plus the time away from my job. The plan was that I would take the shots weekly for about three months, then it would be every other week for a while, and then eventually every month. But after about the tenth week I had deteriorated so badly that when I went in for my weekly shot they gave me a cane.

Things continued to go downhill. Over the next few years, my ankles became so badly swollen the doctor began talking to me about a wheelchair. I had nodules on both elbows, and was in a lot of pain. I stayed on the gold but moved from one anti-inflammatory medication to another, staying with each one until I developed the inevitable reaction, then moving on to something else in the same family.

Friends told me about different things they had heard of that were supposed to help arthritis, and in particular I began to be careful about what I ate. I eliminated chocolate, processed meats that contained a lot of animal fats and gristle like hot dogs and bologna, sugar—I kept hearing about new things to avoid, and I'd cut them out of my life. None of this seemed to have any impact whatsoever, and I kept looking for something new, something that might help me.

And that's how I happened to be looking through the paper one day when I saw a story about a gorilla. The gorilla had serious arthritis, and a doctor at the National Hospital had cured him. I thought to myself, "If this Dr. Brown can do that for a gorilla, I should think he could do something for me." So I picked up the telephone.

The lady who answered at the Arthritis Clinic told me there was a waiting list of somewhere around six months. I thanked her, and hung up. I'm a salesman, and I know how to get past the receptionist in just about any organization I've ever seen, so I called again at a few minutes past five, and Dr. Brown himself answered the telephone. When I finished talking with him, he told me to come in the next day.

I think the thing that decided him was hearing that I was on gold. He told me he was very much opposed to gold, and that he could help me with the arthritis. He outlined in very exact detail what he planned to do for me, and then afterward he gave me a written copy of everything he had said. I told him I wanted to think it over, but that I'd let him know in a few days.

My next stop was George Washington Hospital, where I showed Dr. Brown's paper to the rheumatologist who had been treating me from the onset of the disease. He looked at Dr. Brown's plan for a moment or two, and a little smile came to his face. He told me he knew Dr. Brown, and that he liked him a lot and respected him. He also said he knew of Dr. Brown's theory. He made it clear to me that he did not personally oppose the theory, but he said the problem was that it had not been proven. Finally, he said, "Something tells me you're going to try Dr. Brown's treatment anyway, Mr. Williams, regardless of whatever I might tell you."

I tried to analyze what it all meant. There was nothing mean or disparaging in anything the doctor said; in fact, the tone was positive and friendly, and I felt a little bit as though I had discovered a secret which the doctor already knew but still couldn't acknowledge. I decided that was my answer, so I said, "I'm going to give Dr. Brown's treatment a trial of six months. But if it gets me into trouble and I have a lot of pain, I want you to promise that you'll take me back as a patient. And by the same token, if it seems that after six months I'm getting better, I want you to do a full series of tests and take X rays so you can tell me if the improvement is real or imaginary."

The doctor agreed, and we parted on good terms.

I went over to the Arthritis Clinic and started Dr. Brown's treatment. There were no injections; everything was oral. I expected the results to take a long time to show, but within no more than three weeks the improvement was astonishing. The swelling started to go down, I was able to move around without hobbling, I got rid of the cane, and I felt better than I had felt in years.

What also happened was that my medical expenses dropped from $140 a week, which is what I had been paying for the dangerous drugs that didn't work, to about $35 a month for safe medicine that did. I've had a long time to think about why the medical establishment refuses to accept Dr. Brown's proof, and I have to admit that those numbers keep coming to mind as an important part of the answer. Rheumatoid arthritis is a big, big business.

I've been in treatment with Dr. Brown for the past four years. The pain has disappeared, my spirits have risen, and the swelling that threatened to put me in a wheelchair is now so minor and infrequent that I have no sign of it for as long as a year at a time. I have started my own company in the computer business, something I could never have done in my previous condition.

I wasn't the only one to make a career change. Before the agreed-upon six months were up, I got a letter from my original doctor. It said an opportunity had come along and he was moving to another city. I have since learned that he is no longer practicing as a rheumatologist, and is now a pediatrician.

CHAPTER 7

Connective Tissue

Connective tissue makes up one-third of our body weight, most of it in the form of collagen, which is the protein substance of the white fibers of skin, tendon, bone, cartilage, and nails. Collagen plays an extremely important role in the life of our joints. It is the principal component of the synovium and the plasticlike cartilaginous pads at the ends of our bones that protect the skeleton from grinding itself to powder. And it is the stuff arthritis feeds on.

For the student of arthritis, collagen has some other interesting properties—and in some important respects it is similar to its enemy, the mycoplasmas. You can see the most dramatic of those similarities if you remove the collagen from the skin of a pig. The most likely way for you to extract it is in a form that looks like cotton, in long, fibrous strands. If you put that cottony substance in a test tube and dissolve it with dilute hydrochloric acid, it goes into a solution. Next, put the solution through a filter that withholds all cells. What you now have is a filtrate that looks like pure water and, considering how it was made, would seem to be as free of living matter. But all you have to do is add a touch of table salt to recreate the long, fibrous strands of its original form.

Because this procedure has filtered out all cells, we know that the reconstituted fibers cannot be living matter. What we have instead is a natural plastic that can come and go; like mycoplasmas, collagen can change its state, traveling in and out of the visible world.

COLLAGEN AND AGING

When people get old, the reason they become wrinkled is that the connective tissue between the cells is washed out and the absence of the collagen creates furrows, like mountains and valleys.

When people get rheumatoid arthritis, they appear to age in this same way, but prematurely. The reason is the same, although with arthritis the collagen between the cells is washed out artificially by the active inflammatory process.

Some years ago I read that Colonel Earl Ashe, head of the Armed Forces Institute of Pathology and one of the country's great physicians, had given a speech in Texas in which he said that the cells of the body are immortal, and that the aging process is due to changes in the connective tissue. It was a good line, one that used hyperbole to make an important point. I ran into Ashe some months later at a medical meeting, and I congratulated him on what I had read. He knew that my whole career had focused on connective tissue—what makes it weak and what allows it to become strong again. He smiled when I shook his hand. "I thought of you when I said it," he said. "I knew you'd like it."

If physicians and researchers can find a way to turn off the process that keeps the collagen weak, it will become strong very quickly. The arthritic process keeps the collagen bathed in toxic substances, much in the same way that flame under a test tube can keep the contents unnaturally hot. If the heat is taken away, nature automatically regenerates that connective tissue. People with rheumatoid arthritis always look older than they really are. When they go into remission, the connective tissue begins to regenerate and fill up the gaps, so they automatically look years younger. And they feel a lot younger, too.

TOXINS AND TISSUE

If you look at the thighs of patients whose knees are inflamed with arthritis, the muscles appear thin and wasted and the patient has difficulty rising from a chair or going up and down stairs. The reason for this condition is the same in the muscles and skin as in the joints: the toxic substances generated in inflamed tissues in the knee run up the leg through the lymphatic system and in the process weaken the connective tissues, primarily the collagen supporting the muscle cells. The muscle fibers themselves are not affected, and when the knee inflammation is arrested the collagen reforms and the muscle strength returns. Only if the cause of the inflammation in the joints can be reached and the inflammatory toxins arrested does the collagen have a chance to regenerate. The muscle fibers automatically fill out because a lot of the thinness is due to the loss of connective tissue. Even more importantly, the muscles begin to work again at what an engineer would call their design levels, as the supporting structure of the connective tissues is gradually restored.

Rheumatoid arthritis is a problem of the connective tissues. The inflammatory reaction—where the antibody and the antigen meet—takes place within those tissues and nowhere else. The antigen originates from the mycoplasma and comes out of a cell or on a cell, and the antibody circulates around the system until they clash on this one battleground, producing the toxicity (the formation of proteolytic enzymes) that is so damaging to those tissues.

And what is the substance of those toxins? It can be a mixture of a number of different components: proteolytic enzymes, perhaps a little histamine (an allergy-producing substance), kinins, kallikreins—a whole variety of irritants.

The clash between antigen and antibody in rheumatoid arthritis is the same as the conflict that occurs when you have a runny nose from hay fever or irritated bronchials that constrict from asthmatic allergies; a similar substance is released, causing the observed reaction.

In the case of arthritis, the release of those toxins is damaging, but the damage is not necessarily permanent. If the collagen weakness remains unabated, the body senses that the afflicted tissues might lose their structural integrity and split apart. For that reason, nature reinforces the silk of collagen with the burlap of scar tissues, accounting for the nodules and scarlike swellings in areas of marked inflammation. In cases where the inflammation burns out completely, much of that scar tissue will be absorbed and replaced once again by collagen.

CHAPTER 8

Barbara Matia

A little over eleven years ago, a patient came to me from the Cleveland area without a referral. Her doctors in Ohio had placed her on anti-inflammatory drugs and the antimalarial drug Plaquenil, which can be very dangerous. Fortunately, she decided to try our program before they had given her gold shots or cortisone. From a clinical point of view she stood out for two reasons: her arthritis was raging and was as bad as any I had ever seen—yet there were no visible signs of the disease.

Barbara Matia had been misdiagnosed for years, and even after the arthritis was finally recognized in the face of extraordinarily positive results on her tests, the severity of her case had been completely missed by her doctors. She had been misunderstood through most of her life because no diagnosis of any significant illness had been made until a year or so before she became my patient. Even after her diagnosis, she remained the victim of appearances; her family and friends were equally unable to grasp the seriousness of her illness because she had no crippling or deformity to show for it.

Barbara's battle with rheumatoid arthritis has been very difficult, but it is not unique. Millions of rheumatoid arthritics have had to suffer through disappointment and hopelessness because their disease, like Barbara's, has been misdiagnosed, misunderstood, and mistreated; they have had to battle doctors, well-intentioned friends, and even family to gain the respect they deserve as very sick people.

It took over three years of antibiotic treatment for Barbara to turn the corner and begin unraveling the layers of allergic reaction in her tissues. As she improved, she set herself a goal: to learn why such great resistance to the infectious theory of arthritis had developed in the medical establishment, and to do what she could to eliminate that impediment to the benefit of others suffering from the same disease.

Barbara's quest, which began in 1982, has taken her deeply into Congress, the Administration, and the National Institutes of Health. She has lobbied in support of appropriations to fund infectious research, and with others whom she has enlisted in her cause has testified numerous times before House and Senate subcommittees with oversight responsibilities for NIH funding. Her mission became even more urgent and personal when her thirteen-year-old daughter developed rheumatoid arthritis.

Barbara Matia persisted long enough to see the pendulum finally swing back to a long-overdue reevaluation of the infectious theory of rheumatoid arthritis. Her crusade has made a difference.

HER STORY

When I was five years old, I had an inoculation against measles and suffered a violent reaction. I still remember it vividly. I was in bed for days, my legs and arms so swollen I couldn't see their original shape, and my body was covered with welts. The reaction made me much sicker than the disease would have. I was told that it was caused by an allergic reaction to the inoculation.

I had allergies from the time I was born. My mother had to

get a special formula because I couldn't drink regular milk, and when I graduated to table food I was so allergic to it that I had to eat a single item of food, such as peas, for an entire month before adding another item to my diet.

Three or four years after the measles shot, around Christmas when I was about nine, I again became extremely sick. There was a terrible pain in my jaw, not like a toothache but back in the mandibular joint, as though something had broken; I had a stiff neck, ached all over, and was constantly exhausted. I was afraid I'd miss Christmas, so my mother told me to lie down on a couch in the living room where I could still be a part of what was going on. A wonderful neighbor who we called Grandma Russell came in at least once a day and rubbed my shoulders, and I'll never forget her for it.

My mother took me to our family doctor and then to the Children's Hospital at the University of Pittsburgh. The hospital doctors told her that "debris" had gotten into my saliva glands, and that was what caused the pain in my jaw. They told her not to worry, that it would get better by itself.

Eventually it did. I went back to school, and even though I was constantly weak and tired, my family had done everything they could do and none of us believed there was anything seriously wrong. Later, when I was in my teens, doctors also detected anemia, and it was a condition that stayed with me for years despite repeated attempts to build up my red cell count. But anemia is a common childhood problem, and isn't all that serious. We all knew there was really nothing the matter with me.

One other recollection from those early years is the beginning of a condition that stayed with me into adulthood. At about the same time as the incident with my jaw, I noticed that my skin had become extremely dry and flaky. There were even times when my fingertips would crack and bleed, and my body felt raw. A dermatologist started me on a lamp treatment to help bring out the oils in the skin, but it didn't help. Another aspect of the same condition was that all through my childhood I never perspired; my sweat glands simply didn't work.

What was happening, of course, was that the same disease that caused the arthritis in my jaw was attacking my skin and dissolving the collagen. But lots of people have dry skin; it was nothing to worry about.

Despite the fact that I occasionally had to leave school because of weakness, fatigue, and headaches and frequently had to go to bed after school before I could begin to do my homework, I never thought of myself as someone whose lifetime fate was to be sickly or a cripple. Partly this was because there were no external signs of my arthritis, and the condition went for years without being recognized or treated. Besides, I always had my share of successes in student activities and hobbies, particularly sewing and design.

One day when I was fifteen, I went out to help my mother in her garden behind the house. She had been hard at work for a couple of hours, but ten minutes after I started I was back on the couch in the living room, trembling with exhaustion. I can remember thinking how strange it was that she could keep on working for hours at a time; I thought she was remarkable. I now know it was the high humidity that brought on my weakness and exhaustion.

I lived in the Pittsburgh area with my family all through primary and secondary school, then went away to Illinois for college. At the end of my sophomore year the terrible pain suddenly returned to my jaw, this time spreading to my ears and throat and accompanied by extreme weakness and fatigue. Once more, despite two weeks in the college hospital, no cause could be found for my symptoms. The pain subsided again, but from then on it was always with me, sometimes just beneath the surface, waiting to break through.

In many ways, the absence of any outer signs of my disease was the hardest part. My most vivid memories from all these experiences are not just of the pain and fatigue and weakness, but of the terrible embarrassment I felt about my condition. No one likes to be frail or exhausted all the time, yet with the best of intentions my friends and relatives were constantly saying, "Oh, Barbara, you're always so tired and you sleep so much," as though the condition were within my control and commenting on it would help me to change.

My academic focus shifted at the end of the second year in Illinois, and I enrolled in the Fashion Institute of Technology in New York City. The "Oh, Barbara"s followed me as my New York roommates picked up where the people back home had left off. The comments didn't have much effect; my fatigue only worsened. I found myself looking forward to the short periods, some only ten minutes at a time, when I would be able to lie on my bed and rest. My last year in New York saw me back in the hospital, this time with pains in my legs and knees, and again with no diagnosis.

Perhaps there was another dimension to all of the things I went through during those years that eluded me at the time and only became apparent when I began to get better. I gradually developed a strong determination. It may not have been very evident to others during those long periods when I was so weak and tired, but I felt so inadequate, so "not with it," that I had to keep driving myself just to get by. People with arthritis live in a world of healthy people, and they don't fit into that world unless they learn to push themselves hard and to cope. If they ever get cured, they become great survivors. That's the one thing arthritis is good for.

Somehow I finished school, and on graduation I accepted an offer to join the executive training program of a department store in Cleveland, although I had never been in that part of Ohio before. One day, after I had been on the job for just a few months, the china buyer in the store asked me if I wanted to go with her to a Young Republican Club meeting. I was so tired by the end of the day I just wanted to go home and get into bed, but she talked me into it. It was that night I met the young lawyer who became my husband.

Looking back on it, if there was anything remarkable about our engagement, it was how few opportunities it gave my husband-to-be to learn about me. He was just starting with a law firm and often worked around the clock. After he brought me back from a date he'd go home for six hours of sleep, then work another fifteen-hour day. Meanwhile, I'd sleep approximately twice as long as he did, go into my own job for an eight- to ten-hour day, and return to my apartment completely exhausted. He had tremendous drive and energy. The only way I could compensate was by being very organized.

I became the buyer of lingerie and the demands on my organizational skills increased as the weakness and fatigue began to get worse and the problems with my jaw and neck became more frequent as well. I went on buying trips to New York, where it was expected that we would all work long hours and then be available for dinner engagements with the manufacturers. I sometimes made excuses why I could not stay out for the dinners and other entertainment and took advantage of every possible minute of rest. If the late sessions proved unavoidable, for example, I would make advance arrangements to have nothing scheduled the next morning until half past ten, although everyone else started at nine. When I pushed myself too hard, the end point was always that I would become ill and then collapse.

Even today, the fear that motivated that organization has stayed with me. I still cannot relax enough to rely on having energy when I might need it for a crisis, and I try to plan every move to assure that few crises arise.

The pain in my jaw became so intense in Cleveland that I was unable to chew, so I decided my dentist might be able to give me help where the doctors had not. He looked at my mouth and told me my teeth were out of balance. I spent months going back to him again and again as he tried to bring them back into proper alignment. I spent an enormous amount of time and money but it did no good at all.

The condition was so painful that all I could tolerate eating was milk shakes and soups. I went to a major Cleveland medical center. They looked for everything from mononucleosis to cancer, and I tested consistently negative. Then again, gradually, like the tide, the pain began to recede on its own for a time.

Bob and I were married in 1969, and almost immediately he noticed my unusual fatigue. It annoyed me when he brought it up. I was still working hard at that point, but I could hardly blame my high-pressure job; there are probably few professions in the world more stress-filled than the law. So I told him that the only reason for our different energy levels was that he came from a high-energy family, and not that there was any failing on my part.

I stopped working in 1971 in anticipation of starting a family. I can remember all the things I wanted to do with my free time once I was finished working. We bought an old house in Cleveland with the idea that we would be able to fix it up while we were waiting to start our family, but I became pregnant right away. Our renovation plans fell by the wayside.

I was exhausted for the entire nine months, and of course I explained away the fatigue as a normal side effect of the pregnancy. Once the baby arrived, I simply shifted the blame all over to him; when Doug was six weeks old, an uncle called from Texas to say he was coming to visit us, and I told Bob I was too exhausted from caring for the baby to cook dinner. Bob is solution-oriented. We had a take-out Chinese dinner. But looking back on it, it seems incredible that I could go on denying that there was something very wrong with me.

Bob took me just as I was, and remained sympathetic and supportive. He had come to accept the fact that I required about twice the amount of sleep that he did, and that I ran out of energy far sooner. On days when I felt all right, which still happened frequently, I worked as hard as I could to catch up with the chores that had lapsed when I didn't. I think this helped Bob to see that I wasn't lazy and that there must be a real problem when I told him I felt too tired or ill to move. On days when I couldn't work, I never discussed with him what I hadn't been able to do, and he was so wrapped up in his work that he didn't ask me about how I spent my time when there was nothing to show for it. All I could handle was taking care of Doug and maintaining some household responsibilities; that soon came to be all Bob expected of me.

Nearly two years after Doug was born I became pregnant again, although this time we had not planned it. I love children, and I was delighted with the news. If I had been healthy, we probably would have had four or five. But I wasn't healthy, and this second pregnancy was even more exhausting than the first; I slept much of the time, and for most of my waking hours I was extremely sick to my stomach. A month after Bethany was born I felt worse than ever.

We had a neighbor who had a baby at the same time I did, and I looked out the window one day and saw her cutting the grass. I thought at first my eyes were playing tricks on me, and I couldn't understand where she ever got the energy. But I didn't seriously question why I didn't have as much energy as she had.

As time passed and my condition didn't improve, our internist put me in the hospital for more tests, which were followed by the familiar refrain: they showed nothing of real substance except the usual anemia. This time, however, there were a couple of minor footnotes: there were some signs of inflammation in a small portion of my intestine—perhaps mild ileitis, he thought—and other indications of a low-grade infection. Neither was enough to explain my condition. He prescribed a sulfa drug to clear up the infection, whatever it might be, and sent me home.

For the next several months, I felt better than I could recall since my first days in Cleveland. I had more energy, the pain in my jaw was less bothersome, and my whole outlook improved. When the doctor took me off the sulfa drug, the weakness, fatigue, and pain crept right back into my life.

I dragged myself back to the internist; by this time he seemed to be as frustrated as I was. He suggested that the weakness and fatigue might be related to my blood sugar, and decided to run a test for hypoglycemia. It was one of the most unpleasant procedures I can remember, and seemed to last forever. The results were abnormal, but not enough to tell him anything useful, so, in the absence of contrary evidence, the doctor decided to blame my problems on the female condition; his medical conclusion from all this diagnostic testing was that I was suffering an unusually lengthy case of postpartum blues.

One day I was carrying Bethany across the backyard and my knees became so weak that my legs went out from under me. I protected her from the fall, but the event was terribly frightening to me, and as soon as I got back into the house I called Bob. He couldn't understand what it was all about. "Are you hurt?" he asked.

"No, and neither is the baby," I said.

"Then what's the problem?"

"I fell down," I said. "My legs gave out and I just collapsed."

"Lots of people fall down," he said, and I could sense the frustration in his voice; he couldn't understand why I was calling him. "I'm glad you're both all right."

That night I told Bob that I was certain there was something physically wrong with me, that I couldn't wait any longer, and that if the doctor I had been seeing couldn't help me, then it was time to look elsewhere.

Bob took me seriously. He went back to the internist and told him he didn't want to hear another word about postpartum depression or any other "psychological stuff" until every possible physical explanation had been explored. The internist decided to put me back in the hospital for more tests. The hospital ran my blood through workups I had never heard of. A needle was driven into a bone and a sample of my marrow was extracted. And this time, at long last, the result was different.

We were introduced to a hematologist who told Bob that I was suffering from one of three diseases: leukemia, lupus, or rheumatoid arthritis.

One of the procedures he then ordered was the latex fixation test, which is the standard method for confirming a diagnosis of rheumatoid arthritis. I had taken the test several times in the past, and although I knew that a rheumatoid factor of 70 or 80 would have been serious, the previous results had shown no factor at all. This time they stopped the blood analysis when my readings passed 10,000 and the numbers began to run off the chart.

So I finally knew that I was suffering from a real disease and that I had it in an extremely acute form.

At first, all I could think about were the things I had felt over the years since my early childhood but had never been able to identify or prove. In one degree or another, either explicitly or implicitly, people had dealt with my symptoms as though they were my fault. I thought back on almost an entire lifetime of being misdiagnosed, misinterpreted, misunderstood. Now, for the first time, what I had was a serious, tangible illness, although it was still something the rest of the world could not see.

The rheumatologist to whom I was sent for treatment didn't look at things exactly the same way I did, and my feelings of exoneration were short-lived. He suggested, because the condition was so severe, that there had to be something else on top of the rheumatoid arthritis that made my body react with such fury. Looking back, it's not too hard for me to understand why he took that stand. A rheumatologist who has not been trained in the infectious theory of the disease and who is observing a patient with no outward signs of a severe case of rheumatoid arthritis, such as crippling, would want to explain the patient's weakness, fatigue, depression, and extreme pain in terms of some additional medical problem. He showed no appreciation for what I was suffering, and he told me in the most matter-of-fact way that I would have to learn to live with the disease, as though I hadn't been doing just that for the past twenty years. He told me that he couldn't hold out any hope for the future, that the course was always downhill, and he started me on twenty aspirins a day.

If I was terribly depressed when I went to see him, I was twice as depressed when I came out. When I asked for facts or details about the disease, he reacted as though he resented the question. In time, I realized that his responses followed a pattern. Instead of giving me any information, he first admonished me for not accepting my condition, then usually followed up by raising some psychological issue as though the spectacular activity on my charts was entirely a product of my mind. I very quickly came to feel betrayed by the person I had first thought would rescue me, and those feelings soon reached the point where I disliked our visits very much.

Moreover, instead of getting any better, I soon wound up in bed, unable to do a thing.

My faith kept me going, and I took each day as it came, one at a time. We got full-time help in the house to do the laundry, the cooking and cleaning, and to take care of our one-year-old daughter and four-year-old son. As soon as I woke up in the morning, I could hardly wait to finish my few brief conversations with Bob, the children, and our help so I could get back to sleep. I slept sixteen hours a day, and some days right around the clock. It went on that way for month after month.

The pain and fatigue were the first part of the disease that I had to deal with, and then I began to experience more of the muscle weakness that had made me fall in the backyard with Bethany; my legs were unreliable, and my arms wouldn't do some of the things I asked of them.

Then came the intense pain.

Now it was in my entire skull, and I took Percodan every four hours to relieve the hurting. Then the pain began to spread, surfacing for a time and then disappearing at different locations throughout my body. My spleen became enlarged, my liver became enlarged, my adrenal function became depressed, and my heart muscle was affected, causing severe shortness of breath; it wasn't until later that I learned the disease attacks every tissue or organ that depends on the blood, including the entire length of the arms and legs, not simply the joints. By the time Bethany was a two-year-old, the arthritis had taken control of my entire body from head to toe. I lay in bed feeling as though I had been run over by a truck.

A nurse came in to put hot packs on my joints every four hours. They were so soothing I hated to feel the heat leave them, and I lived for her visits. Sometimes the flares of pain would last for hours and hours, then would suddenly come to an end, and I would feel enormous relief.

When it became obvious that aspirin wasn't doing the job, the doctor put me on Plaquenil. He said that Plaquenil could cause blindness and that I would have to be checked regularly by an ophthalmologist. He also told me what lay ahead, setting out the whole program for the typical arthritic: when I could no longer take Plaquenil, I would go to gold shots, and when the gold shots wore out I could move on to cortisone, and so on and so on. He told me that some arthritics go into remission after the first year or so—not because of anything the doctors do, but because of the disease itself; we both knew that I had already had arthritis for a lot longer than a year.

Bob resigned himself to my disease. He didn't want to hear about the pain, because there was nothing he could do about it, but he was absolutely committed to doing anything he could to help me with every other part of my life.

One day, Mary Jean Rice, a caring, cheerful woman from our church, came to our house to visit me. She brought several articles written by a rheumatologist at the Arthritis Institute of the National Hospital for Orthopaedics and Rehabilitation, outside Washington, D.C., who had made amazing progress with arthritis. She told me that Dr. Thomas McPherson Brown had treated her for several years, and although she still wasn't cured, her arthritis was much better than it had been when she first sought his treatment.

I liked Mary Jean and I was sure she was telling the truth as far as she knew it. But I found it very hard to believe something so exactly the opposite of the picture painted by my own rheumatologist, that this disease of unknown cause was actually an infection and that it could be reversed. That night I showed the articles to Bob and asked him what he thought.

We had already gone through a lot of other remedies—

mostly special diets and teas—that we had read about in newspapers and magazines. He said he would read through the papers I gave him, but that he had serious doubts about it. "If the Cleveland medical establishment doesn't have the answers, no one does," he said.

Meanwhile, I read through the material myself and became more and more interested. A couple of nights later I told Bob I wanted to go to Washington to see Dr. Brown. His response was guarded. He told me we couldn't afford to travel all over the country every time we read there was another cure for arthritis, because we were seeing that kind of story about once a month. A couple of days later I called the Arthritis Institute anyway. The woman I spoke with told me the earliest available date to see Dr. Brown was a year away. "All right," I said. "I'd like to make an appointment."

I told Bob that night. He was upset that I had made the call, but with the appointment being a year away he figured he had plenty of time to change his mind.

The passing of that year had just the opposite result. I was able to stay on the Plaquenil, but instead of getting any better I spent most of the next twelve months in bed, even to the point where I had to be served most of my meals there. We both deliberately avoided thinking about the future. It was a terrible year; I lay in bed, watching everyone around me functioning normally and leading productive lives, and we saw my own life slipping by, vanishing, with nothing to show for it but pain.

My appointment was in September, which meant that I would have to endure another Cleveland summer. The hardest time with arthritis is when there are changes in the barometric pressure, especially when accompanied by rises in humidity. Cleveland's weather is constantly changing, so I was in a state of nearly continuous flare.

Bob was very fortunate in finding great support from several of the other lawyers in his firm who, with the natural skepticism that lawyers apply in their quest for the truth, assisted Bob in analyzing our medical options. When the notice arrived to remind us that our appointment was coming up soon with the Arthritis Institute, one of the things they did was to make inquiries within the medical community in Cleveland about this Dr. Thomas McPherson Brown. What they found out was that no one seemed to know if there really was anything to Dr. Brown's approach—some suggested that it was unproven, and others went so far as to say it was medical quackery—but there was unanimous agreement that his credentials were impeccable. And even if his treatment didn't work, antibiotics weren't dangerous and there seemed to be very little risk.

Bob remained unconvinced, but I felt I had nothing to lose in trying this treatment program. Bob said that if I were determined to see this Dr. Brown, he wanted to accompany me to the meeting, and he made me promise in advance that I wouldn't begin treatments until he and I had both talked it over and agreed. That sounded just fine to me: Bob was a lawyer, and he knew how to ask for information and analyze the answers. I trusted him completely and greatly valued his judgment.

When the time finally came for my appointment, I was too sick to fly, so Bob made up a bed for me in the back of our station wagon and we drove to Washington.

We arrived late in the afternoon and checked into the National Hospital. I was shown to the room I was to share with a woman from Alabama who was also visiting Dr. Brown for the first time. Bob and I were told that he would be coming by that evening to meet the new arrivals.

My roommate and I immediately started comparing notes on our disease. She told me that she had just come back from Europe and that she had been given gold and cortisone shots by her rheumatologist back home to get her through her trip. I remember thinking to myself, how on earth could she get through Europe with arthritis? I had barely been able to make it from Cleveland, Ohio.

Looking back on it, that conversation was my first real indication of how isolated I had been and how little I still knew of the disease that dominated my life. I got rheumatoid arthritis without knowing where it came from or how long I had it, I was told what medicines to take with no promise that they would work or that I would have any kind of a future, and the only real advice I ever got was simply to live with the disease and cope as I was able.

When Dr. Brown arrived that first evening, he spent a long time with us. I was so tired from the trip that after a while I began to lose track of the conversation. Dr. Brown was explaining what was known about the arthritis disease process and telling Bob all he had learned about how the infection can be treated and eventually cured. Two of the things I heard were that it would take two and a half years of treatment before I would "turn the corner," and that I would get worse before I started to get better. I couldn't imagine feeling any sicker than I already felt, so that part didn't hold much fear for me. And compared to the length of time I had already been sick, two and a half years didn't seem like a very long time.

Finally, after answering a long series of questions by Bob, Dr. Brown said good night and told us he would start both my roommate and me on tetracycline therapy the following morning. Bob looked at me and smiled, and I smiled back; that was all the discussion we ever had about whether to go ahead. He turned and shook Dr. Brown's hand.

Later, when the lights in the room went out, I put my head back on the pillow and wondered what it would be like to feel well again. For the first time since I had been diagnosed, I was given hope; it was a moment I will always remember.

I spent three weeks at the National Hospital on that first visit. Near the beginning of my stay, a nurse came by one morning and told me she was taking me down to therapy. I was so weak I needed a wheelchair, and after that first session I pleaded with her not to take me down again. Dr. Brown came to visit me frequently, and he told me in one of our early conversations that I had one of the worst cases of arthritis he had ever seen. It may be hard for someone else to understand, but it meant an awful lot to me that he said that;

all of my life until then, I had almost nothing tangible to point to—no wounds, no sores, no scars or deformities to match the way I felt, no evidence of the terrible thing that was raging inside my body.

Bob stayed with me in Washington the entire three weeks. His firm has an office there, so he was able to work during the day, visiting me at the hospital in the morning and evening. In some ways, the trip seemed to do him more good than it did me. Until then, neither of us had a clear picture of what was happening to me, and the lack of a pattern or of any hope had been terribly defeating to us both. Now it all changed. Bob is very focused and has great energy, and as a result of what he learned from Dr. Brown I could see him responding to my disease as though he were lining himself up on a target, aiming at the first ray of light at the end of a long tunnel, filled with hopefulness and enthusiasm.

Although I was every bit as resolved as Bob, hopefulness and enthusiasm are not in the arthritic's arsenal. One of the first things Dr. Brown asked me when I saw him alone was how I was handling my depression. No one had ever spoken with me about that side of the disease before, and I was immediately defensive. "I'm not depressed," I said. I had not grown up in a world where people permitted themselves to think that way.

Dr. Brown smiled patiently. He knew from long experience that arthritics are reluctant, at the beginning, to discuss with their doctors any symptoms except pain; in fact, with anyone else most arthritics learn not to talk about their condition at all. "Depression is a part of the disease," Dr. Brown said gently. "Nobody can have rheumatoid arthritis without being depressed."

"All right," I said. "I'm depressed all the time." I was startled to hear myself say it. The mycoplasma wasn't the only thing that had buried itself way below the surface; I had been fighting to suppress everything, including my own feelings.

"Well," he said, "you'll find that when the rest of the disease goes away, the depression will go, too."

Later, somewhat guardedly, I told Bob what Dr. Brown had told me. To my surprise, Bob nodded and said he thought I had been depressed for a while. It was not something we had ever discussed before.

My reactions to the intravenous treatments of tetracycline were every bit as unpleasant as Dr. Brown had predicted. He told us that the mycoplasma releases toxins when it is attacked, and the more deeply it is entrenched, the worse the toxic flare. He kept me on aspirin as my anti-inflammatory drug. The best part of having him visit me every day was that he was able to keep me informed about what was happening as it took place, interpreting my reactions; he actually made me feel fortunate that the treatment was causing so much discomfort, because that was one sure sign that it was attacking the disease.

After a short time on the intravenous therapy, an oral form of the same antibiotic was added to my medicine so that I would be able to continue using it at home. For the whole three weeks, Bob asked more questions than Dr. Brown had ever heard before, and by the time we left the hospital he knew more about the infectious theory of arthritis than the average rheumatologist. Dr. Brown had also armed us with a realistic understanding of the difficult road ahead, and having that kind of map would make it a lot easier for us to get where we were going.

When we returned home, all I could do in an entire day was take a shower, and even that was an agony of exertion and pain. We even had a physical therapist come in to carry out a massage program that was intended to help remove the toxins more quickly. At times I became discouraged about the treatment, but then Bob would keep me going. It was as though we had completed a circle: I was the one who persisted long enough to get us to the hospital, and it was Bob who held us on our course once the therapy began.

For a while, we returned to the hospital in Washington every six months. As Dr. Brown predicted, I was getting worse and worse.

We decided to take a vacation in Phoenix. This wasn't a decision we made because I felt better. We had heard from one of Bob's law school classmates who also suffered from the disease that Arizona's climate was about the best in the United States for arthritics, that it was stable and dry, and that the barometer didn't keep rising and falling as it did in Cleveland. We flew out, but the trip was too much for me; as soon as we got there I had a flare-up that put me in bed for a week.

The second week was much better. I was able to sit outside and spend a little time with the children, and Bob and I even spent a few early evenings together on the porch. By the end of the month, although it was an effort, I was actually able to go out with him to dinner. My spirits began to lift as well.

When we returned to Cleveland, it was the middle of the usual rainy springtime, and I went right back to bed. Although neither of us wanted to face a hard decision, the comparison between how I felt in Phoenix and how I felt in Cleveland was compelling.

Bob was a rock. He told me it was not nearly as hard as it might have been; he could finally understand the disease, he knew what was happening, and he knew it would eventually end. He was absolutely wonderful with Doug and Bethany.

That was the hardest part for me during this period of my life—the feeling that I wasn't able to take care of our children myself. Looking back on it, they probably didn't miss very much because I was there for them almost all of the time, to talk with them, answer their questions, and keep them company—probably more than if I had been healthy and spent my days pursuing the normal responsibilities of a housewife and mother. But sometimes when I was really suffering and Bethany got up on the bed and asked me to help her color, I knew that moving a crayon would make me hurt even more, and I couldn't do it. Even when I wasn't particularly in pain, playing a simple game with the children would wipe me out and I would have to rest for two hours just to recover.

It would probably take a psychologist and an accountant to figure out whether the children gained more than they lost by having a mother in my condition during those years, but there was a big part of me that said I was letting their lives as well as my own slide by. The guilt fed on the depression that went with the disease.

The issue of where we lived started me questioning the other priorities in our lives. I became very disturbed that we were so tied to Cleveland, particularly by Bob's new partnership in his law firm and by his family's active involvement in local politics. I talked with Bob about this and told him one night that I really wanted to move to Phoenix, at least until I had "turned the corner" on Dr. Brown's treatment program. He didn't say anything, and by the time we went to bed he was still quiet and seemed to be troubled by our conversation. The next morning he got up early, and when I said good morning to him, he told me we were moving to Phoenix.

He told his partners that day. He explained that we had to get away from Cleveland's weather patterns until I started to improve and that we expected this to take another two years. The head of his practice area asked him not to be too quick to leave the firm until he had a chance to explore an idea he had. The idea was that the firm would open a one-man office for Bob to continue his Ohio law practice from Phoenix. The firm would send his work to him and Bob would complete the written aspects of it in Phoenix, returning to Ohio as necessary for meetings with his clients. Bob's partners were wonderful, supportive people. We still had the idea that once we got through the stage of my disease where I "turned the corner" as Dr. Brown had predicted, we would move back to Cleveland, so instead of selling our house we rented it.

We moved in September, five months after our vacation visit. As we drove out of town, we thought about the friends who had brought meals to us or had watched the kids and been such important parts of our lives. In particular, we thought about our friend and neighbor Hilde Clark, who accepted our version of what was happening because it made sense to her as a former nurse. She cooked for us, cared for our kids, filled in for canceled housekeepers and shared her love and faith. We would not have made it without Hilde.

Every seven years or so, Phoenix has a rainy cycle, and, of course, it coincided with our arrival. We found a woman to come in and take care of the house and children, Bethany went to nursery school, Doug entered the first grade, and I spent the next several months in bed while Bob studied for his Arizona bar exam.

I continued going to Washington at the six-month intervals, and I could feel myself getting closer to the long-awaited corner that Dr. Brown had promised. I was no longer getting worse. Then, almost without realizing it, I was getting better.

At first, it showed up in small ways. I started thinking beyond myself, and I began to do things for others. Instead of spending all my time and energy on coping with the disease, I was able to do things like fix dinner and even run small errands outside the house, perfectly ordinary things that were now a source of delight. I still couldn't do the dishes, but if I washed the clothes one day I could fold them the next, and it was so thrilling to me that I couldn't imagine ever complaining about having to do the laundry again. I found more energy to do things with the children. Gradually, I added more and more responsibility to my life.

The biggest step toward recovery was feeling well enough to drive the car again after two and a half years. And the biggest shock I received was seeing how grocery prices had gone up since I had last shopped.

Even with the trend toward improvement, the flare-ups were just as strong as before, and every time they happened I would feel for a time as though I had been sent back to the beginning. The problems this created for the scheduling of our lives were still among the hardest parts of the disease; we had to live day by day and hope to be able to get through whatever lay directly ahead. It was terribly embarrassing to make a plan for a week later, only to cancel when the day came because I had no muscle strength and was exhausted and in pain.

But, undeniably, I was getting better. Each six months, I would compare the results of my various blood tests with results from previous trips, and the progress was measurable. There was another kind of comparison that went on during those same trips that was even more encouraging: I would meet other patients who were on the same visitation cycle as I was, and they kept looking healthier, more cheerful, and more energetic every time I saw them. It was as though the movies of their lives were running backward in six-month installments, and every time we went to Washington they were six months younger than they had been the time before.

What it all meant, I realized one day, was that we had all turned our various corners and were now advancing toward unbelievable recoveries. Our lives were being returned to us. We were on the road back.

In 1982 I went to Washington for my semiannual treatment and checkup, and someone told me that Dr. Brown had been invited to testify before Congress. I was pleased to think that at last the infectious view of arthritis was getting the attention it deserved, and that evening, when he returned to the hospital, I asked him how it had gone. He said that he was glad to have been asked to testify, but that he had no idea what result it might produce.

The next week, back in Phoenix, I asked Bob what he thought would come of Dr. Brown's testimony, and he said, "Nothing. Nothing at all." He thought the problem was too immense.

I was unwilling to accept that possibility. It seemed beyond comprehension that a program which has been developed by a doctor whose credentials are second to none and which has helped over ten thousand sufferers of arthritis was not being accepted by the nation's medical establishment. I decided to do whatever I could to help make that happen.

I have known what it is like to live without hope. I know what it is like to be given hope. And I know what it is like to have a disease reversed and to be able to live a full life again.

Today I live a rewarding, happy life as a wife and mother,

and I spend substantial amounts of time working toward getting federal funding for research into the infectious causes of arthritis.

The disease that brought me to this work is almost gone; Dr. Brown told me when I first met him that it would leave the way it came, and the only remaining symptom is an occasional flare-up and pain in my eyes. I work hard, my depression left me long ago, and I function as well as anyone else on a normal amount of sleep. I am very near to the end of the long road back to total recovery.

The more I have worked at influencing public opinion about the true nature of rheumatoid arthritis, the more I appreciate Bob's view of the size of the problem. But I made a promise to myself that afternoon eleven years ago when Bob and I arrived at the National Hospital, and I have tried to keep it. The promise was that if the treatment worked—if it could relieve my pain and give me back my energy, my family, and my life—I would find a way to return the gift.

CHAPTER 9

Symptoms and Diagnosis

Barbara Matia's experience is not unique. For the victim of rheumatoid arthritis, tangible evidence of the disease may not show up in a form that can be readily identified until it reaches its acute stage, with nodules at the joints and even disfigurement. But the physician who sees the patient in time can recognize the first symptoms far earlier, perhaps as much as a year and a half before these external physical changes occur.

WHAT DOCTORS TELL PATIENTS

The first sign of rheumatoid arthritis is not pain, but fatigue with no good reason. The history of the fatigue and of what the patient does about it often follows a predictable pattern. As a rule, when the victim realizes that he or she needs more and more sleep, the logical response is to see a family practitioner. Several tests are done, and the doctor usually reports that there is no apparent physical cause for the condition. He then asks the patient, "What's bothering you? You seem to be under a great deal of tension."

The physician is on pretty safe ground. Every person who ever visited a doctor is under some kind of stress; that's the nature of modern living. The patient thinks about it for a moment, and then acknowledges that the doctor is right. In this brief exchange, for no other reason than that the doctor can't figure out what's wrong, some of the responsibility for the symptoms has been subtly shifted to the patient. The doctor nods in affirmation and says, "Well, you'll be all right. I think that's all it is."

One of the other symptoms of rheumatoid arthritis is depression. That takes a lot of the fight out of a person, so at this point, many patients meekly get up and go home. Others are unwilling to be dismissed that quickly, and they ask the doctor if there's anything he can do to make them feel better and restore their former energy. Sometimes the physician prescribes shots of vitamins, but as a rule he says no, that things will get better by themselves.

The next step, before there is any visible change, can be an unexplained anemia. This is something a little more tangible for the doctor, who now tells the patient he knows the cause of the problem and sets about curing it with shots of vitamin B-12, iron, and sometimes folic acid.

But the hemoglobin doesn't rise as it should, and the doctor asks the patient more questions: "Are you taking the medication I've given you?" and "Is there something you're not telling me?" The patient says yes to the first and no to the second, but the questions have served a secondary purpose: the seeds of uncertainty have been planted, and the patient wonders if the real root of the problem is something he is doing that he shouldn't, or not doing that he should.

Another preliminary symptom of rheumatoid arthritis can be unexplained weight change, and this takes two forms. In some cases, people who are slight of build will lose weight; when accompanied by severe fatigue this is often a precursor of the painful phase of the disease. In other cases, the patient is already overweight, and as the disease progresses the patient's weight increases, despite efforts to control it. We have observed this same phenomenon of weight abnormality in patients with other connective-tissue diseases, including scleroderma and lupus. But as any of these diseases go into remission, both extremes begin to move nearer to the mean; patients who are too thin start to gain, and those who are obese find that their efforts to reduce are becoming more productive.

ALTERNATIVE DIAGNOSES

It usually isn't long after these various symptoms appear before the patient begins to get some joint pain. There is still no visible external evidence of change, but the pain is a new symptom and calls for another trip to the doctor. At this stage, and even as long as a year later when the pain combines with some of the early signs of disfigurement, many doctors are still unwilling to diagnose the condition as arthritis. Favorite alternatives are sciatica, bursitis, lumbago, and synovitis; the apparent rationale is that any curable disorder is preferable to one that is not.

By the same token, if the doctor understands that rheumatoid arthritis can indeed be cured, then he also recognizes that all of these delays are detrimental to the patient and can greatly extend the degree and duration of treatment.

PROVING THE PRESENCE OF THE ARTHRITIC INFECTION

If a patient comes to me with the earliest of these symptoms and nothing external yet shows, I start off with a test for the mycoplasma complement fixing reaction. It was through this means that I recently confirmed my suspicions about the eleven-year-old daughter of a woman I had been treating for several years.

The daughter was always tired and wasn't doing well in

school, and I suspected a combination of fatigue and depression, the classic early signs of rheumatoid arthritis. Like most children, she was unwilling to admit to much of anything that would aid in her diagnosis. This was partly because of a natural tendency for children to hide their feelings from adults as they seek to establish their own identities, and partly because of a lack of experience against which to make useful comparisons about how they *should* feel. Depression is particularly hard for adolescents to handle or for doctors to recognize; it doesn't show in children the way it does in adults, and is mixed in with a lot of psychological and physical changes that are normal parts of growing up. As a rule, it manifests itself as indifference. The child doesn't get out and play with others of the same age but is more inclined to read, watch television, or simply withdraw.

Despite the mother's insistence that her daughter probably had arthritis, because that was the way her own had begun when she was more or less the same age, the girl's doctors were not inclined to accept a lay diagnosis, especially when their own standard tests for the disease were negative. But when a sample of her blood was sent to our laboratory, the far more sensitive mycoplasma complement fixing reaction showed a high degree of activity, and I immediately wrote to her mother that the test, combined with the girl's other symptoms and her history, gave strong evidence of rheumatoid arthritis infection. We started her on a course of antibiotic therapy, and because it was still relatively early in the course of the disease, she picked right up and did very well.

At the end of the summer, however, my young patient hit a slump. Her spirits dropped again and she showed some of the earlier lethargy, though not as strongly. Her parents were prepared for this to happen. The mother knew from her own long experience that there are three flare periods in early stages of the treatment for rheumatoid arthritis: September, February, and May, the months in which the barometer is least stable. At those times, a doctor has to reassure his patient that it is normal for the recovery to slow down and even lose some ground for short periods, but that the slump won't last and that as the treatment continues the dips eventually stop occurring.

Up to the time of this writing, my patient, now fourteen, has had rheumatoid arthritis for three years and has been in treatment for two. Her energy levels have risen, her symptoms of depression have vanished, she gets along on a normal amount of sleep for a girl her age, her earlier outgoing nature has returned, and her grades in school are up to honor levels.

The mycoplasma complement fixing reaction by which she was initially diagnosed is a test for the antibody that develops in the bloodstream in response to a mycoplasma infection. In order to do the test, it is necessary to have strains of mycoplasma available in the laboratory. So far, no such strains are obtainable from commercial sources, so the Arthritis Institute propagates and stocks its own supply. However, it would be a simple enough matter for a pharmaceutical manufacturer to produce such a product. As mycoplasmas finally gain recognition as the cause of rheumatoid arthritis, laboratory testing kits should soon be appearing on the market.

ARTHRITIS AND TEMPERATURE

There is one other symptom involved in rheumatoid arthritis, but it is a subtle one and easy to overlook in a diagnosis. That is a very slight temperature elevation. Lyme disease is a form of rheumatoid arthritis that in its early stages presents itself differently from other types, and a pronounced fever is one of its more dramatic features. (Lyme disease has played a key role in improving the medical community's understanding of rheumatoid arthritis as an infectious illness, and is discussed in detail in Chapter 16.) With other rheumatoid forms, the temperature is usually just a fraction above normal, and the few tenths or a single degree of abnormality will often escape detection. If the temperature is measured with an electronic thermometer, however, in a doctor's office or a hospital, the slight elevation can be seen easily. It isn't the response to an invading germ, as is the case with Lyme disease, but rather is a reaction to a substance which the germ produces. This small temperature difference is one of the most exact objective indicators of profound fatigue, and often of the depression that goes with it. Once the patient has begun treatment with an antibiotic, the temperature flattens right out at normal.

This small rise in temperature is less significant as a guide to diagnosis than it is as a further proof that rheumatoid arthritis is an infection, and it is a sensitive indicator to the effect of treatment. I often make use of it when I do patient rounds at the hospital. If I see from the chart that the small fever has disappeared, I'll tell the patient I am glad to see he or she is feeling better. It's a great trick, and until I explain it, the patients often feel I have a special diagnostic gift.

HYPERSENSITIVITY

One of the central concepts for understanding how rheumatoid arthritis works is that of the "sensitized host." Hypersensitivity is really the same thing as an allergy, but it occurs in a system where it doesn't produce a standard allergic display, such as hives or the rash from poison ivy.

The human body is made up of three sections. The ectoderm includes the skin, part of the eyes, the lungs, and part of the trachea and esophagus. The entoderm is the gastrointestinal tract and its attachments. The mesoderm includes the connective tissue, bone and cartilage, muscles, nerves, blood and blood vessels, the lymph system, and the remaining glands and organs.

Each of these sections is separate in the embryo, and although they combine in later stages of development, each retains its own unique status all through life, each reacting differently and each the target of various allergies, although the entoderm can include some ectodermal and some mesodermal features.

It has occurred to me over the years that the mesoderm is primarily the focus for bacterial allergy, while the ectoderm is more the target of chemical allergy. Obviously bacteria are chemical as well, but I am referring more to such irritants as ragweed, dust, and smoke. The distinction is not complete, because we can get hives from a vaccination or from a food reaction, but the three sections do react differently even to the same stimuli.

Mesodermal allergies don't show on the surface, and because of that we don't generally call them allergies; for that matter, for a long time we didn't even call them hypersensitivities. But as time has passed, I have become convinced that one of the major pathogenic components of rheumatoid arthritis is the fact that the mesoderm is reacting in a truly allergic sense to the agents for which it is the particular target. These agents include mycoplasma, streptococcus, brucella (the agent of undulant fever, which gives rise to arthritis), tubercle bacillus, and others.

NODULES: THE CLASSIC HARBINGER

The most pronounced and classic symptom of rheumatoid arthritis is the nodule, which appears at the joints as the first external evidence of arthritic disfigurement. Because this is so widely recognized for what it represents, some victims of the disease are actually relieved when the first rheumatoid nodule appears; now, at last, the patient has something tangible to take to the doctor. Nodules usually arise at the site of some injury, such as a sprain or bump, and although it is possible to have one or two without necessarily having arthritis, it is likely that all such nodules are the result of disease activity at the site.

Nodules are unlike malignant lesions that keep on spreading, however, and they can come and go. Sometimes a patient will detect one on an elbow or wrist and make an appointment with the doctor, only to discover that the nodule has receded and perhaps even disappeared by the time the appointment is kept. Or it can vanish in one place and reappear later in another.

The most likely explanation for these nodules is that they contain fibrous tissue that forms in a skein around the small lesions where the mycoplasmas are located. The tissue is a protective response by the body to contain the infection and keep it from spreading. If the mycoplasma antigen stops coming out for some reason, either because the body's defense puts it down for a while or a medicine suppresses it, then the scar tissue surrounding the germ is no longer needed and the nodule goes away. The process by which this occurs is one of natural attrition; cells are periodically replaced, and if the cause for defense is no longer there, the body will remove the old cells without sending in new ones.

THE ROLE OF STREPTOCOCCUS

People who have the most rheumatoid nodules are frequently the ones who have had a streptococcal infection, perhaps in childhood, and in whom there is evidence that the streptococcal antibodies are still present along with the mycoplasmas. The drugs for streptococci are not the same as the ones used for mycoplasmas. If I detect streptococcal antibodies, I will combine an antistreptococcal approach with the treatment for the mycoplasma at the outset, and once the streptococcal level has been lowered, I will focus the attack more precisely on the mycoplasma.

The standard treatment for streptococcus is penicillin or one of its many derivatives. Penicillin has no value in treating the forms of rheumatoid arthritis that are caused by mycoplasmas—the vast majority of such cases. (They do work on the form known as Lyme disease, however, which evidence indicates is caused by a spirochete bacterium.) Conversely, the tetracyclines aren't as effective as penicillin in treating streptococcal infections. The problem in using penicillin-based antibiotics is that they tend to create drug allergies after a certain amount of time, so there is an incentive to limit the duration of their use. After a short term of treatment with penicillin derivatives, the rheumatoid nodules tend to disappear in patients who have the history of streptococcal infection.

HOW RHEUMATOID ARTHRITIS WORKS: A CONCEPTUAL VIEW

There are lots of other variables that have to be considered in assessing a patient's condition and monitoring the effectiveness of treatment. Most of them are subtle and some are highly elusive. But all of them have in common that they are totally incompatible with the methodology of double-blind controls, which up to now has been the universal technique by which treatments for rheumatoid arthritis are evaluated. Even the smallest of these added factors calls into doubt the reliability of the results achieved in treating the basic disease.

Over the course of the half-century in which I have studied rheumatoid arthritis, bit by tiny bit I have developed a medical design based on a conceptual view of how rheumatoid arthritis works. That view is extremely important in the decisions I make about the basic approach to treatment and in the fine tuning as that treatment progresses. In my mind, I constantly see what is going on inside a patient's body, much as I suppose atomic physicists envision the mostly invisible electrons and protons with which they work. Any physician who treats rheumatoid arthritis must develop this same conceptual view of the mechanism as a frame of reference for the process he is managing, both in formulating short-term tactical responses and in designing an overall strategy for each patient.

OTHER TESTS

The mycoplasma complement fixing reaction is just one of several tests I order when I am seeing a patient for the first time. I also routinely ask for a complete blood test which measures the hemoglobin, red blood count, white blood count, differential white cells, and other factors. White blood cells, which are the body's first line of defense against disease, are divided into several types: lymphocytes, monocytes, granulocytes, basophils, and so on. These differential white cells can shift when under attack, and if rheumatoid disease is very active the lymphocytes go up.

That rise in lymphatic activity is an excellent gauge of the progress of treatment for rheumatoid arthritis. But long before I took advantage of that useful feature, I became interested in lymphocytes for another reason: they increase during rheumatoid activity, and the polymorphonuclear cells do not. Polymorphonuclear cells are the ones that increase during appendicitis, lobar pneumonia, or staphylococcal or streptococcal infections, for example, because it is their job to go after regular bacteria that invade the body. Lymphocytes are quite different; for the most part, their tasks are related to the immune system, particularly the creation of gamma globulins. They are activated by viruses of all kinds. They are also activated by the cousins of the viruses—the mycoplasmas—against which they generate antibodies.

When I first observed this phenomenon many years ago, I began to look at diseases other than arthritis in which the lymphocytes were high. I saw that they were also very elevated in rheumatic fever, as well as in a great many other rheumatic-type illnesses such as lupus and scleroderma. I began to monitor their levels during treatment of patients with tetracycline in order to confirm that the lymphocytes were indeed performing the role I envisioned. Those studies showed such an exact cause-and-effect relationship that I now use the same tests as a barometer of the patients' progress toward recovery. If the physician wants to get a quick preview of what the laboratory technician will see under the microscope, all he has to do is touch the lymph nodes in the patient's neck; swollen glands indicate high lymphocyte activity.

Sedimentation

Another simple blood test that tells the physician a lot is the sedimentation rate. It was found long ago that when blood is put in a tube with an anticlotting substance, the cells settle to the bottom of the tube in a predictable and diagnostically useful fashion, a reversal of the way cream rises as it separates from milk. A line forms in the tube. Above that line is the straw-colored component of blood which is the plasma, and at the bottom are the red cells. The line itself, a thin layer just above the sinking bottom portion, is made up of the white blood cells. The speed at which these cells settle out of solution correlates with the rate of activity of the rheumatoid process—how "hot" it is.

The doctor or technician measures the distance the blood settles in the tube in one hour. Sedimentation rates vary by gender: a rate of 30 or below is normal for a woman, and 15 for a man. The reason for this 100 percent difference is probably related in part to the fact that the blood sedimentation rate rises when a woman menstruates. Typically, with active rheumatism the readings will be ten points higher than normal in either sex. Sedimentation testing is not entirely specific for arthritis—any inflammatory reaction will produce the same results—but it provides a good diagnostic indicator and it is also useful in monitoring the effectiveness of treatment if given every six months or so.

Bentonite Flocculation

Every incoming patient is also given a Bentonite flocculation test and a latex fixation test. Both use foreign substances that react with certain globulins that produce a kind of anti-antibody called the rheumatoid factor. This anti-antibody is a second line of defense for the body in fighting off the arthritis infection; when it tests positive the condition is more dangerous and more difficult to treat because it means the source of antigen is surrounded more vigorously by an additional wall of defending substances. The tests vary in that Bentonite flocculation is more delicate and will often give positive results when the latex test is still negative. Bentonite is also sensitive to other infections and allergies, however, while the latex test is more specific to rheumatoid arthritis. A second reason we give them both is that by the time the reaction shows positive on latex as well, we have one more clue to how far the disease has developed.

SMAC

Another standard requirement when I accept a new patient is the SMAC (for Sequential Multiple Analyzer Computer), a total blood appraisal including different chemical tests. Alkaline phosphotase, for example, if way out of line, indicates that the liver isn't just right, and creatinine, a waste product excreted only in the urine, provides clues to kidney function. Cholesterol and triglycerides are also tested. The SMAC also shows albumin levels of the blood, which are depressed if arthritis is very active and come back up to normal as the patient gets better. Other chemicals that change in the presence of arthritic activity are calcium, phosphorus, sodium, potassium, and uric acid; some go higher and some lower.

In addition to being comprehensive, the SMAC is also very accurate because it is automated. This is a distinct advantage over human measurement of these same minute quantities, a procedure which varies widely from lab to lab and from test to test, even on the same source. The SMAC makes it possible to compare test results obtained on opposite coasts, which previously would have been nearly meaningless.

The importance of accuracy and reproducibility in such tests can be seen in an exercise I did some years ago in connection with uric acid. At certain levels uric acid is associated with gout, which is easily confused with rheumatoid arthritis. When I was at George Washington University, because I was very skeptical about the reliability of manual testing, I sent a blood sample from one person to four different laboratories for a uric acid determination—and I got back four entirely different results. In one case the reading was a clear indication of gout. In another, it showed the patient was entirely free of it. The automation of these tests is a great step forward; without reproducibility, their results would be worthless.

Joint Scan

If the patient is admitted to the hospital, the next diagnostic procedure is a joint scan, using a gamma camera to view the way in which technetium 99, a rapidly degradable radiopharmaceutical, concentrates in the affected areas. The so-called "hot spots" where the concentration is heaviest provide a graphic, dynamic, and objective measure of the degree of arthritic activity of the joints. When viewed in sequence over the course of a prolonged treatment, two or three annual scans also make good visual reports on the progress of therapy, a feature that is as uplifting to the patient as it is informative to the doctor.

Kunkle Test

Another standard diagnostic procedure is the Kunkle test, a special gamma globulin measurement of how hard the body is fighting against the mycoplasma. Gamma globulin is a combined globulin that is the precursor of certain types of specific antibodies in the blood. If a person is suffering from typhoid fever, for example, the body calls on the gamma globulin pool to make antibodies against the typhoid germ. If somebody in the household has hepatitis and we want to avoid getting it, we will go to the doctor for a shot of gamma globulin because it contains a number of different antibodies that have built up in the donor's body over the years, including, possibly, some antibodies to hepatitis.

X Rays in Diagnosis

As a final diagnostic tool, if they seem to be indicated, I also order X rays. The principal area in which X rays are helpful is the hips, which are different from most of the other parts of the body in the ways they react to rheumatoid arthritis. Hips can become badly damaged even when the rest of the body is improving. This is largely because of the way they are formed and connected to their arteries. The circulation in the hip is different from that in the femur in the legs; it comes through the socket of the hip into the head and down to the neck. The shaft of the femur, on the other hand, is circulated by vessels that go down the side of the leg and then into the bone. People who are very active physically and who are likely to damage their hips, such as dancers or high hurdlers, are also likely to damage the circulation of the head or femur, especially in cases of dislocation. If that happens, the femur shows signs of dysfunction when the rest of the leg is fine, because the socket of the femur doesn't necessarily conform with the state of affairs that pertains to rheumatoid activity. It is hard to know whether this circulatory liability is also a part of the pathology of arthritis. But whether it is or not, the problem is not nearly as serious today as it was a few years ago, thanks to advances in hip prosthetic technology and new surgical techniques.

The primary purpose of all these tests, beyond aiding in the diagnosis, is the establishment of a baseline. It is also worth mentioning that the purpose of the blood tests we order during the course of treatment differs from the purpose of such tests in virtually all other forms of rheumatoid arthritis therapy: we are measuring the effectiveness of our treatment in curing the disease, not how quickly the patient is being poisoned by his or her medicine.

CHAPTER 10

Bob Matia: Living With an Arthritic

I think the first indication I had that something was wrong was before we were married, when Barbara told me she had intermittent pain in her jaw—and then, as the result of a fall, the pain increased substantially. The doctors had to wire her jaw, and we all thought it would be one of those things that clear up in a couple of weeks. But ten weeks later the pain was still there.

Then, after we were married, I noticed that if we were out late, Barbara often couldn't get up until ten or twelve the next day. I come from a family where everyone got up early regardless of what time they had gone to bed the night before, and I thought this long recovery period was a sign of frailty. I have since learned a lot about the disease, in particular that this lack of stamina, this low level of base energy, is one of the symptoms and effects of severe systemic rheumatoid arthritis. But of course we had absolutely no idea that was her problem at the time.

I knew Barbara wasn't lazy. She worked extremely hard as a buyer for the department store, and she'd take the stock room apart from top to bottom, then visit four or five of the thirteen branch stores in a single day and meet with salesmen along the way. She was also very disciplined at organizing her life to get the most use out of the energy she did have.

We had other early indications that things weren't right—all related to fatigue and lack of energy—but it really wasn't until our second child, Bethany, was born that Barbara went into a tailspin and the disease began to rage.

After Bethany's birth, but still before we had a diagnosis, there were times when nothing Barbara did made any sense to me. It didn't seem reasonable that she should feel all right at ten in the morning, and when I'd call her at two in the afternoon she'd be in bed. It worked the other way as well; I'd call from work in the middle of the morning and she'd be asleep, and when I called again in the afternoon she was feeling much better. One of the most difficult parts of the disease—difficult for everyone in the family—is its total unpredictability.

I remember one particularly frustrating experience. Before Barbara's problem was diagnosed, we were invited to a dinner party at a partner's house one evening, and when I got home from work on the appointed day—less than two hours before we were supposed to be there—Barbara announced she was too sick to go. I had a clear picture of all the preparations that had already taken place at the house where the party was to be held: the floors were carefully vacuumed and mopped, the furniture dusted and polished, the table was set with fresh flowers in the center; in the kitchen the roast was cooking in the oven and our hostess was starting to prepare the vegetables. I turned to Barbara in a combination of anger and despair, saying, "Why couldn't you have decided this in the morning? Why did you have to wait until the last minute?"

But I knew the answer before she said it: in the morning she had felt just fine. It was all the more frustrating because at that point we still didn't know what was the matter with her.

Arthritis is a real mystery disease. It can be difficult to recognize and diagnose, and it can appear in ways that most doctors even today are not aware are parts of the disease. This unpredictability about the way an arthritic is going to feel is the norm, and the arthritic has no control over when the flares will occur. If the nonarthritic partner doesn't understand those things, the marital relationship can be put to a hard test.

Even after Dr. Brown told us all the ways that arthritis changes one's life, we still kept running into people who would say, "But *that* isn't arthritis. Arthritis hasn't got anything to do with your mood or your energy." Now and then, well-meaning people would come by to cheer up Barbara, to open the curtains and raise the window in her bedroom, telling her that what she needed was a little sunlight and fresh air. They thought they could talk her out of it, that the whole thing was in her mind, and they related her physical condition to what they supposed was her mental attitude. They had it exactly backward. It was almost as though they could not comprehend that rheumatoid arthritis was something that could land a person in bed at such a young age.

Barbara's disease became a serious problem at a point in my career when I was expected to put in long hours and be available at the drop of a hat to any client or partner who wanted my time. The greatest difficulty her illness presented for me professionally was when I had to call my office in the morning and tell them I couldn't get in on time because of the situation at home. And frequently, I stayed late at the office when I really should have gone home.

There was one particularly difficult period during the preparation of a bond issue in which the legal aspects were very complex and the matter dragged on for months. Once a transaction reaches a certain point, it is very disruptive to substitute any of the lawyers in the transaction. Barbara understands that fact of life, but it didn't make any difference to her arthritis. She was at the time experiencing difficulty breathing and was having strong flares of weakness, inflammation, and pain. Day after day, I would leave the house early and return late, too tired to give Barbara the emotional support that she so desperately needed.

The tensions Barbara's illness created for my career would have been a lot worse if it weren't for the support I received from the partners and associates of my firm. They backed me up, filled in for me at important meetings, and spent time helping me weigh choices and find solutions to the many problems, both medical and personal, associated with her disease. Not everyone who is married to an arthritic is that lucky.

Despite all the support, there were times when I asked myself why I deserved the life I was leading. Why should I be the one to have to carry this special burden? On one occasion there was a document drafting session in New York City, and at the last minute I had to get one of my fellow associates to fill in for me at the meeting so I could stay home with Barbara who was in a severe flare at the time. The associate called me at ten one night to ask me a question about the documents, and I can recall my feeling of irrational resentment at his needing to consult with me when I still had a lot ahead of me that night. When the load gets too heavy, people tend to shed the last straw, regardless of how legitimate that straw may be. I should have expressed gratitude instead of annoyance for the work he was doing in my place.

After Bethany was born, I spoke several times with our family doctor about the sudden increase in difficulties Barbara seemed to be having. He was a highly competent and respected physician in his specialty but he did not have the training or experience that would have allowed him to conclude that the symptoms we were describing to him were all parts of the same disease mechanism. Like many doctors educated in the 1940s and 1950s, he was of the school of medical thinking that explained any seemingly unrelated symptoms in psychosomatic terms rather than physical terms. As a result, all these talks wound up at the same place, with him saying that Barbara's symptoms were the result of psychological factors. And he said this based on very limited medical testing, very limited experience with us as a family, and without having requested from Barbara her medical history, which would have indicated a consistent pattern of undiagnosed symptoms from the time she was five years old. I have since learned that arthritics are frequently forced to deal with this kind of reaction.

Finally I went into our doctor's office one day and literally banged my fist on his desk, saying I didn't want to hear one more thing about psychology until we had exhausted every other possibility of a physical explanation. It was a risky move; he was also the doctor to three of the senior partners in my law firm whom he knew socially as well as professionally, and it wasn't hard to imagine that if I offended him enough he might be inclined to make some casual comment to one of them about Bob Matia's grace—or lack of it—under pressure.

"I want you to put her back in the hospital and give her every test known to the medical profession," I said. "This has dragged on far too long, and I don't want to live my life this way anymore."

It worked. He put her back in the hospital, and this time the hematologist came back with a different report: Barbara's blood cell structure indicated that we were probably dealing with leukemia, lupus, or rheumatoid arthritis. Our doctor then ordered further tests to determine which of these it was, and the results for rheumatoid arthritis went right off the charts.

Barbara's response to this new information was subdued because she had an aunt with arthritis and she knew something of what lay in store. But I was elated: I wasn't going to lose my wife to a fatal disease, and more than that, I felt tremendous relief on finally being able to point to a tangible physical disorder that I later learned from Dr. Brown explained absolutely everything we had been dealing with.

It wasn't until a long time afterward that I learned from Barbara how she really reacted to my delight. While all I was feeling was relief, she had to deal with the discovery that her symptoms were part of a real condition that was long-term and perhaps even permanent. I went happily to a golf outing of my law firm with the attitude that it was "only arthritis." The fact was that Barbara still had all the earlier symptoms, and despite the fact that we now knew what caused them, they were getting worse.

But something else happened during this same period that

helped us both. Barbara had asked me before we were married what my religion was, and I had replied by asking her what she wanted it to be. I never had any strong feelings about the religion in which I was raised, and anything that I did feel in those early days had soon vanished in my years in an engineering program. So I was perfectly willing to take on her religion—she was a Presbyterian. And her faith was strong. But the casual attitude on my part soon changed under the pressure of our needs, and I became active in a local Presbyterian church in Cleveland.

I also spent a lot of time in concentrated thought about how to cope with my overlapping responsibilities. In these periods of contemplation, I began to feel the clear and unmistakable guidance of a Supreme Being. And with that new awareness came the beginnings of a sense that our separate and mutual burdens somehow would be made bearable, and that our needs would be answered. That faith is a great victory that has come out of this adversity, and it yielded dividends in our own relationship even before we met Dr. Thomas McPherson Brown.

In addition to my new faith, there was another wonderful gift that derived from Barbara's arthritis, and that was the close relationship which it permitted—or forced—me to develop with our children. Even though Barbara communicated with them and gave them emotional support the entire time she was bedridden, there were periods in their early youth when I was their father and their mother (at least from the standpoint of custodial care); I have often thought that if it were not for Barbara's illness, it would have been easy for me to become so preoccupied with success in business that I would have been neither.

These uses of adversity may be sweet, but they are hard-won. What we went through together contributed more than any other part of our lives to our spiritual growth and to the growth of our characters.

I found it very difficult to discuss Barbara's pain and discomfort with her. I always have tried to be a very positive person, partly because I had found early in life that a gloomy or tense situation can be changed into a tolerable one, and a positive attitude was a way to create a positive environment and often a positive result. Barbara adjusted to living under that kind of constraint. Later on, I learned that it is very common for arthritics to not discuss their pain and suffering with those closest to them, and for the same reason: they have reached a tacit understanding that that part of the burden cannot be shared because it cannot even be understood by someone who has not lived through the same experience.

The arthritic is trapped, too sick to live a normal life yet cut off from the true understanding of the loved ones who are trying desperately to share the burden. To some extent, the trap worked both ways; as long as we were bound together, our lives were governed by the same disease. However, there is one major difference: the arthritic has no choice. Though they never say it, they both know that the partner does.

When a patient on tetracycline therapy finally turns the corner and begins to recover from rheumatoid arthritis, the recovery embraces all aspects of the disease, not just the pain and inflammation. Three years after Barbara began her treatment at the National Hospital, I saw that she was not only emerging from the prison of crippling and pain and depression, but she was also shedding the fetters of self-centeredness. Her body no longer clamored for every minute of her attention, and she no longer hoarded every ounce of energy for her own overwhelming needs. She started thinking again of others, and of giving. And she discovered that as a result of her illness and progress toward recovery she had something extraordinary to give.

The healing of rheumatoid arthritis is usually a long, slow process. The recovery takes place in layers, with a little bit of the disease being peeled away at a time, and in between, the affliction folds down again; when that happened, Barbara would seem as sick as ever. During the protracted reemergence of the real Barbara Matia, the disease continued to play its cruel game of hide-and-seek. But the periods during which

Barbara was herself became longer and longer, and the times when the disease was in control grew correspondingly shorter and less frequent.

As her general condition improved, she kept stretching herself to do more things than she had been able to do before, and frequently she would get caught between the layers of recovery. I recall one night, for example, when we went to a restaurant for dinner. I looked forward to the night out as a break in our routine. But our food had barely arrived when I saw from Barbara's face that she was in a lot of pain, and that she was struggling to keep up a front. I told her I wanted to take her home, that I couldn't enjoy myself knowing what the effort cost her. She said she wanted to stay, that it meant a lot to her to be able to do this for us. We stayed.

The two most difficult times for a husband and wife are when the arthritic spouse is just going into the disease and when he or she is coming out of it. In between, while the illness is at its worst, nothing much changes and neither partner has to continually learn new roles. When Barbara was sickest and without hope of recovery, we knew we had to hire nurses, we knew we had to get someone in to take care of the house and the children, and we knew we were faced with an unending path of pain and suffering—but there was a predictability in our lives, and even though it was a tragic predictability, at least we could rely on it. But as she began to get better and the situation changed almost daily, we found our relationship changing right along with it, erratically, even wildly, and often painfully.

Anyone can understand the letdown that goes with arriving home in the expectation dinner will be ready, only to discover it is not because at the last minute one's partner became too sick to prepare it. It's harder for people to understand that it also can be a letdown to come home with a bag of groceries and a dutiful plan for fixing dinner because one's spouse is sick, only to find that she is standing in front of the stove and a completely different dinner is ready to go on the table. Barbara was reluctant to give up her responsibilities even when she was too sick to perform them, and I was reluctant to give them back when she began to feel well again. Each of us secretly resented the other for this perceived usurping of responsibilities.

This recovery period is also difficult for friends to understand, and as a result the arthritic becomes adept at covering up the bad periods. People's view of the healing process is that when recovery begins, it continues unabated; there aren't supposed to be wide swings in how the patient feels, and certainly not all in the same day. To friends and bystanders, this can look like game-playing. That's where the cover-up comes in: arthritics learn to smile and say they are feeling fine when they are really sick. Going through the layers of this disease in either direction is not recommended for people who cherish routine.

One of the things that couples eventually discover in living through the disease is that many of the hardest problems they face with rheumatoid arthritis are problems they would also face, albeit to a lesser degree, without it. Arthritis obviously has some special difficulties all its own, but the hardest parts usually come from the magnifying effect it has on the little things in the relationship, on the strengths and weaknesses that are so basic and so taken for granted that they are seldom examined or changed except under some such extreme duress. Under the arthritic lens they become immense, and the disease forces both partners to face them. Some people flee from the vision, and the marriage ends. Despite our failings, on balance Barbara and I were blessed with faith and determination. The disease used us both, but we used it as well—to reshape what we were at the start, and to improve our life together.

CHAPTER 11

Depression and Other Psychological Parameters

The organic aspect of rheumatoid arthritis—the deformity, crippling, and pain—is obvious to everybody. When psychological problems appear, as they inevitably do, many physicians regard them as a forerunner of the disease or an aspect of stress that would be natural with any chronic, progressive problem. It has not been generally recognized that these psychological symptoms are actually a component of the disease process itself.

"IT'S ALL IN YOUR HEAD"

When patients go to a doctor for treatment of their arthritis, they seldom mention these psychological problems. In some cases, the patients don't believe they are related to the disease. In other cases, the patients are afraid the doctor will think the psychological symptoms are causative and will request that the patient seek psychiatric care before undertaking the treatment of the disease. These patients are used to being told that the problem is "all in the head," and they don't want to add any more fuel to the fire. Many arthritis patients have sought psychiatric care but found that it did not help their arthritis, despite some mental relief.

We have found at the Arthritis Institute that the psychological symptoms of arthritis are indeed a component of the disease process, and when the disease goes into remission, these symptoms clear up. Of all the aspects of successful treatment for which the patient is grateful, by far the most important is relief of the psychological problems which are a part of the disease. Despite their importance, however, they are the least recognized by friends, family members, associates and physicians. Severely depressed rheumatoid arthritics have long since stopped talking about their disease because they know that nobody wants to hear about it, including their doctors, so they live with it inside of them, and the pressure of suppression only makes things worse. What the patients feel when those psychological symptoms finally depart is enormous relief and gratitude.

As noted, there are a number of psychological or invisible physical symptoms that usually precede the development of the rheumatoid disease expressions by a year or longer. When confronted with the characteristic unexplained fatigue, the doctor's first suspicion is of anemia or low thyroid function. Usually all tests prove to be negative at this point. If anemia does exist, it is not generally corrected by simple measures.

Other such symptoms are an inability to concentrate as well as usual and a loss of interest in avocations and hobbies that were previously sources of enjoyment. The short-fuse syndrome is very common in this phase, and in many patients who are ordinarily very calm and well controlled it is totally alien to their normal personalities. The annoyances that the patient expresses are usually justified, but not to the degree the patient exhibits. After a particularly energetic outburst, the patient is usually chagrined, but only when it seems too late to easily correct it.

DEPRESSION IS ORGANIC

By far the most disturbing of any of the psychological symptoms is depression. Generally it comes in very short episodes, lasting from just a few hours to a few days. When the depression hits, it can be devastatingly severe, but is seldom suicidal. In the more than forty years I've been observing the behavior patterns of the rheumatoid arthritic patient, I've known of only two who committed suicide at the height of one of these depressive episodes; both were in psychotherapy at the time of death.

A FAMILY DISEASE

Family members, like doctors, usually attribute the arthritic's depression to the pain and distress that go along with the disease process, and they don't recognize it as a symptom in its own right. Those in close contact with such patients urge them to go out and do something different, to become active, and this only aggravates the situation. As these episodes of depression are generally short, it is far better to leave the patient alone until the condition passes.

It is extremely important for family and close friends to recognize the nature of this depression and that it is a part of the disease. In that respect and in many others, arthritis is a family disorder; this recognition is the best treatment the patient can possibly receive, and it is equally healing to those who give it.

Even in intimate family life, however, those who live with the patients are seldom able to share fully in the feelings of the arthritic or to help through the standard methods of encouragement. At the National Hospital, the first thing many new patients experience is a feeling of tremendous relief at being able to talk about their arthritis with those in the beds around them, people who are interested and who share their experience. People have a great need to express themselves about things that weigh heavily on their lives and to prove to themselves that their afflictions are not unique. They also need to learn that people actually get better, that they are able to recover from a disease that everyone else has told them is supposed to go progressively downhill. Husbands or wives of arthritics are victims of this same depression, only at second hand. They are constantly trying to cheer up their mates, trying to coax them into some kind of activity that will take them out of themselves, and they are constantly being thwarted by a mate who is often too depressed to move. I have had many patients over the years whose marriages have held together only because the time was taken to carefully explain the role of depression and how it can affect relationships. And I have had many others whose marriages had already ended.

PARTNERS

There are two kinds of partners of rheumatoid arthritics. One type of husband is very supportive of his wife and will do anything for her—and instinctively leaves her alone when she's depressed, not trying to jolly her out of it, because he knows it doesn't work. He watches for the moments when the sun begins to shine and then takes her out to enjoy it. Arthritics have sudden ups and downs, either with pain, fatigue, depression, or other psychological symptoms, and the mate must learn how to take advantage of the highs without becoming ensnared in the lows.

The other type of mate fights the disease, and part of that fight takes the form of denial. Arthritics are truly not responsible for the mood swings created by their affliction any more than they are responsible for the pain and crippling. Depression will not go away simply by willing it to stop.

Families need a great deal of help in understanding and coping with the disease. The majority of the patients who have these multitudinous problems look quite well, and they are unable or unwilling to say how they really feel, knowing full well that others don't want to hear discouraging things. Besides, to discuss how you hurt is boring to others.

The psychological difficulties associated with arthritis are thought to be caused by an immunologic defect, and not by a personality flaw in the patient. Learning the proper response to a depression which has this organic base does not necessarily require the skills of a psychiatrist; it is mostly a matter of common sense. It is a great step forward when the patient learns that his psychological behavior pattern is part of the disease process itself and that it will improve when the cause of the disease is recognized and treated—and that it will not improve in any lasting way when symptoms alone are treated.

STRESS-PROOFING THE ARTHRITIC

An important step the treatment of any rheumatic or collagen vascular disease problem is the removal of any unnecessary stress. It is useful for the husband and wife to appear together for the interview with the doctor and to tape the conversation for further reference and understanding at later stages in the course of treatment. Rheumatoid arthritis is complicated and its treatment embraces some elusive concepts which are often particularly difficult to retain when the patient's memory is below par as a result of the disease. One of the concepts which the patient should hear and record is that long-term treatment of the basic problem will restore the memory to normal functioning.

After all these years of treating rheumatoid arthritis, I am convinced that the most important aspect of the disease is, surprisingly, not the pain but the way a person feels about himself. The lifting of depression and the regaining of interest, the desire for accomplishment, the improved mental functioning, all seem to give the patient a new life. The process of premature aging comes to an end and the patient realizes there is a great deal left to live for.

There could be no understanding of the relationship

between the psychological parameters and the disease process itself until it was possible to reach the source of the problem. It seems clear from our experience that the basic problem is not addressed by any of the symptomatic treatments. On the contrary: In the long run, the traditional treatment methods allow the fundamental disease process to progress under the cover of symptomatic relief.

We have also found that psychological parameters are of vital importance in determining the distance covered on the road back. These psychological factors have not been generally recognized or employed as they should be, as important milestones for measuring and marking therapeutic accomplishment.

CHAPTER 12

John Doe, M.D.: The Doctor as Patient

This case history has been disguised at the subject's request. Dr. Doe, a gerontologist, lives and practices in a Virginia suburb of Washington, D.C.

I had my first symptoms of rheumatoid arthritis in the fall of 1984. They began as neck pains, and at first I suspected the cause was the position of my head on the pillow during sleep. Although they were worst in the mornings, they pretty well disappeared after an hour or two, and there were some days when I didn't have any pains at all. But after they had persisted intermittently for about a month, I went to my family doctor for a test of my RA factor. (The RA, or rheumatoid factor, is a relatively recent discovery and has proven to be very valuable in the diagnosis of rheumatoid disease.) The result was positive, and he sent me to a rheumatologist.

By the time I kept that second appointment another two weeks had passed, and the pain had spread to my right shoulder. Part of my practice as a physician involves physical exertion in dealing with elderly patients, and I found the condition was beginning to interfere with my ability to help them on and off the table and to assist them in changing positions during examinations. However, I saw the rheumatologist in the afternoon at a time when my pain wasn't bothering me, and he said to me, "Well, Doctor, you look just fine," and gave me a prescription for ibuprofen, an anti-inflammatory analgesic which had already been prescribed by my family physician.

A week later my shoulder and neck bothered me so badly I called the rheumatologist again. His answering service told me he had gone on vacation, and I left my name for the doctor who was taking his cases; that doctor, who knew nothing about me, didn't bother to return my call for three days, and by then I was in agony. When he finally did call, I told him I had gone elsewhere.

Elsewhere was a rheumatologist in Baltimore, referred by another physician from the hospital in northern Virginia with which I affiliate. I told the Baltimore doctor the case was an emergency, because the condition was now making it difficult, and at times impossible, for me to continue my practice. He was so busy he couldn't fit me in until the middle of December, more than a month away, but that was a lot better than being out of town or not returning my call, so we set a date.

At our first meeting he said he wanted to admit me to the Baltimore hospital for further study, and I agreed to a week in early January 1985. I was reluctant, because it meant taking time off from work at my own hospital and required the rescheduling of a lot of my elderly patients who do not take well to change.

By the time I entered the hospital, the pain in my neck had improved noticeably. My shoulder was worse, and there were new pains in one knee and the opposite hip. The study involved a joint survey with whole-body X rays and a full repeat of all the laboratory tests I had undergone earlier. While I was going through this, I noticed that I was beginning to feel light-headed and slightly dizzy, and all my joints were starting to get unusually warm, which I mentioned to the doctor. He wasn't surprised; he told me the tests showed my hemoglobin had dropped from my normal of 12 or 13 to 10 grams and the sedimentation rate was up 20 points to 55. He took my temperature rectally and it stayed normal; only my joints were hot. When the tests were completed, I was sent home with three prescriptions: one for prednisone, one for Plaquenil, and one for a nonsteroidal anti-inflammatory. My life as an arthritic had begun in earnest.

In the months that followed, I never had any fear that I would die from the arthritis, but there were many times when I seriously wondered if I would survive the treatment.

My first problem with medication was a rash which developed all over my body within two weeks of leaving the hospital in Baltimore. I called for a return appointment, but the problem with seeing a successful rheumatologist between regular visits is that the patient has to sit for up to five hours in the waiting room surrounded by chronic-looking patients, and each such journey turns into a day-long expedition. Already, I had sacrificed more of my professional time to the treatment than to the disease itself, and the situation was only to get worse in the months ahead. When the doctor finally saw me, he stopped the first nonsteroidal anti-inflammatory and put me on low levels of another one called Feldene.

Over the next few months, my life was reduced to little more than working, eating, and sleeping. I was recently divorced at the time, and a woman cousin who lives nearby in Maryland often helped with my cooking and drove me back and forth to my appointments in Baltimore. I managed to get to work on my own, but there were days when my wrists were so painful and my hands so weak I was unable to hold the steering wheel of my car and was forced to call in sick. Over the next four months, because of the steroids, my weight increased by fifty pounds, up from a normal 170 to a very uncomfortable 220.

That June I went to work one morning, put in a normal day, and at about two in the afternoon I noticed that my hands were becoming so stiff that I had trouble using them. This was an ominous departure from my usual experience, in which all of my inflammation and stiffness had occurred in the morning, and I decided to head home as quickly as possible;

something really bad was coming, and I knew if I stayed around any longer I would have to be admitted as a patient. I was not eager to advertise my physical liabilities among my peers as I was afraid it might affect my future at the hospital.

When I got to my locker I was unable to open the door and had to ask an intern for help, but then I decided things were happening too quickly for me to take the time to change and I headed out to the garage. Somehow I opened the door to my car, and as I sat behind the wheel I dropped the keys on the floor. After I finally got them into the ignition lock, it took another twenty minutes to turn them enough to get the engine started. My hands had lost almost all of their strength, especially in the rotational motion of the wrist. Driving home was no problem because the car has an automatic shift and power steering, but once I reached my house I was unable to turn the wheel enough to park in the garage, so I pulled over to the curb on the street. It took another half hour to turn off the key, and that much time again to walk up the path to my front door and into the house. Once inside, I went to the bedroom and called my cousin. "I don't know what's happening," I told her, "but you'd better get right over. I can't move."

I badly needed to relieve my bladder, but I knew I'd never make it to the bathroom on my own. I lay back on the bed and waited for my cousin.

By the time she arrived, I had been lying in one position long enough that I couldn't even turn my head. I asked her to call a good friend of mine, an orthopedic surgeon, to get the name of a rheumatologist whom he had recommended several months earlier. I also called Baltimore and talked to the resident at the hospital where my present rheumatologist practiced. I told him I was suffering a severe arthritic attack and asked what I could do. He told me I could drive to Baltimore, but even if I did there wasn't much they could do for me because my regular doctor had gone home; the best he could offer was to give me some Demerol. I decided not to go. (Since I've been sick with arthritis, I have carefully avoided any of the painkillers like Demerol or morphine because of my fear of becoming addicted; the strongest medication of that kind I ever took was Darvocet-N 100, and in two years I didn't use a hundred tablets.)

My cousin dialed the rheumatologist my friend had referred me to, in a Maryland suburb of Washington and much nearer to where I lived. He agreed to see me the next day.

The following morning I was better, but not nearly well enough to go to work or to drive to the doctor's office by myself. My cousin came back at noontime and we drove to the doctor's in her car.

This time the doctor started me off on aspirin, coated to avoid disturbing my stomach, which by now had become sensitive to almost every form of medication. The doctor tried to take me off the steroids, but every time I stopped taking them I became so stiff and inflamed that he had to start me right up again. He then tried tapering my dosage to a low level of five milligrams every day, but it took five tries and six more months before he was successful in stopping the steroids altogether; during each of those failed attempts, I'd be all right for about a week, and then I'd become so stiff again I couldn't move.

But what this new rheumatologist was taking away with one hand, he started putting right back with the other. He began a program of injecting cortisone directly into my wrist joints, and a course of treatment with gold salts. The gold was like mustard in both appearance and effects. I don't know which treatment was more painful. In a short time I noticed that my normally brown hair had started turning red from the gold injections, and I asked him with a certain amount of irony if I were eventually going to become blond. A few days later I received an even more ironical answer when I discovered that the hair on the top of my head had started to fall out.

Besides all that, the gold didn't work. After five months, the doctor decided to try yet another approach and he switched me over to penicillamine.

The penicillamine was a great relief from the gold for two reasons: it was administered orally and didn't require the painful injections, and it worked. The arthritis came under control within just a few weeks, and for the next couple of months I felt terrific. Then one morning as I was shaving I felt something odd on my upper lip, somewhat like an insect bite, and as I looked more closely I saw that I was developing a blister. Within a few days it had spread to the inside of my mouth and cracked down the middle both inside and out; then it started to bleed, and pus appeared at the edges of the lesion.

The rheumatologist decided the blister had nothing to do with the treatment and he sent me to a dermatologist. The dermatologist took one look and quickly agreed; he said the blister was more likely related to the arthritis itself, and he gave me a steroid cream to spread over the affected area. By this time I was becoming certain that the real cause was the penicillamine, but when I suggested it a second time, the dermatologist said he would watch it for a while and if it got worse he would do a biopsy—not an answer that encouraged further discussion.

Shortly after the blister appeared, I began to notice new symptoms in my eyes. I had always been highly allergic by nature, reacting to almost everything from dust to feathers to pollen and all the other known irritants, and as a result I was not unused to having my eyes become red and teary. But this was something new; whenever the reaction started, it would come on like a tornado and I would be nearly blinded by the water in my eyes. I wondered whether it might be stress-related, but I dismissed that idea when I considered that my arthritis was better than ever, I was able to do my job well enough, and my life seemed to be relatively stress-free.

I went to see an eye doctor who told me it was probably just an unusual form of allergy. He gave me some drops to put in several times a day. One morning a week later I looked in the bathroom mirror, and what I saw there belonged in a Dracula movie; my eyes were fiery red. The ophthalmologist didn't have any new ideas and just told me to continue using the drops. But a few days after that I was at work and I ran into an eye surgeon who took one look at me and asked if I had rheumatoid arthritis. When I said I did, he examined my eyes closely and told me that my tear ducts had stopped producing tears, a not-uncommon effect of the disease. He gave me artificial tears, which I applied three times a day.

Meanwhile, I was developing a reaction to the aspirin which the doctor had prescribed in place of the steroids. I experienced dizziness, ringing in my ears, and lightheadedness. The doctor told me to cut down, and after I did I called him back and said I planned to get off the penicillamine as well. I reasoned that if the relatively minor problems with the aspirin were sufficient to cut back, then the far more serious effects of penicillamine were a good argument for quitting altogether.

About two months later I went back for a check-up and found that all the test results had started climbing again. The penicillamine hadn't changed anything; it had merely masked the effects of the arthritis, and now they were coming back to the surface. The doctor told me he wanted to put me back on the penicillamine. I was scared to death of it but, like him, I couldn't see any other choice. I took one tablet, and the next day my lips were completely covered with blisters.

It happened that on that same day, I had my weekly appointment with the physical therapist who had been helping me to work with my affected joints. He took one look at me and said, "You know, you really ought to be seeing Dr. Brown at the National Hospital."

I had never heard of Dr. Brown, and I asked the therapist who he was. He told me about Dr. Brown's treatment, which he said was sometimes described by others as "unconventional and unproven." He said that although they had never met, he saw many of Dr. Brown's patients who were recovering from rheumatoid arthritis, and he was very impressed with the fact that they were all getting better. Without much hope for the results, I called the National Hospital for an appointment and was told Dr. Brown wouldn't be able to see me for six months. I asked the appointment secretary to put me down for the first opening, in June.

I returned to the doctor who had started me back on the penicillamine, and when he saw the new blisters he immediately switched me over to methotrexate. “This is my last one,” he said. “Let’s hope it works.”

“Let’s,” I said.

I stayed on the methotrexate for four months, but when I saw Dr. Brown I stopped and have been on a simple antibiotic ever since.

Dr. Brown warned me of the Herxheimer effect when I began the tetracycline therapy, and although the effect lasted a month I could feel myself becoming better even within the first week. (The Herxheimer effect, described in Chapters 16 and 18, is a reaction to treatment in which the symptoms of a disease get worse at the start of therapy, a paradoxical sign that the infectious source of a disease is under attack.) It was as though I could actually feel what was happening at the cellular level in my body, that the cause of the arthritis was being attacked and destroyed and carried out of my system, and it was terrific.

I have been in treatment with Dr. Brown for only three months, and I have improved immensely. My hips and knees are now in perfect shape and I can walk briskly for the first time in two years; I have more energy, I can exercise more each day, my damaged hepatic function has improved, my eyes are better, and I am returning to health. The wrist joints in both arms were already damaged by the disease before I reached Dr. Brown, however, and this treatment is not going to increase their limited function. I still have a distance to go, but I feel that I am on the road to full recovery.

I wish I had heard of Dr. Brown’s treatment two years earlier, in time to save me the unnecessary suffering, the expense, and the damage to my career and my body which I have lived through in the interim. And I hope by telling my small part of Dr. Brown’s story, I will help the world to get to know him better and save others from my own all-too-common experience.

CHAPTER 13

Arthritis Research: A Brief Overview

Many years ago, particularly around the turn of the century, rheumatoid arthritis was generally considered to be an infectious problem. The reason for this view was that there were a certain number of people who first had kidney trouble, a bad tonsil, or some other infectious complaint and developed arthritis soon afterward. It was assumed that the focal infection was the cause of the arthritis, and that if the focus were excised, the infection would go with it.

FIGHTING INFECTION WITH SURGERY

It was an era in which surgeons moved very quickly to take out all the removable parts that could be a source of infection, such as tonsils, the appendix, ovaries, the uterus, a kidney, the gallbladder—and often the synovial membrane from the affected joints. It was a devastating period for sufferers of arthritis because many of them were on the operating table within a day or two of complaining of the first twinge in a joint. The surgery did have an impact on the arthritic condition. Some patients improved markedly, but the results were not consistent, and many others got worse. As a result of unsuccessful joint surgery, some were crippled for life.

That draconian approach to arthritis quickly turned into unwarranted excess. It went on for ten or fifteen years, until finally, like each of the successive chemical treatments in the modern era, it ran its course. The principal reason for the demise of this particular approach to the disease was the rise of the American Rheumatism Association, which stood as a bulwark against unethical practices and treatments of arthritis that clearly didn't work.

Unfortunately, when this kind of surgery fell into disrepute, the infectious theory was badly weakened as well. The baby, which was perfectly healthy, was thrown out with the bath water.

In the course of many decades of studying the disease as an infection, I have developed a theory for why some arthritics were improved by the surgery. I suspect that when some people got dramatically better after the surgical removal of a localized infection—in the gallbladder, tonsil, kidney, or wherever—it was because they were still in the early stages of the arthritic infection, and their bodies had not yet had time to become violently sensitized against the bacterial antigen. Conversely, those who did not do well after surgery were the ones who had suffered from arthritis so long that they were sensitized by exposure to the bacterial toxins—toxins that had been pouring into the bloodstream for months or years. When the focal area was attacked surgically, it released yet more toxins into the system of the already sensitized host, showing up in the form of a postoperative flare.

STEROIDS AND THE ECLIPSE OF INFECTION

At about the midpoint of this century, the infectious theory went into a steep decline as the conceptual view of the arthritic mechanism took a sudden and unexpected turn. In the late 1940s, a researcher named Philip Hench at the Mayo

Clinic announced several new extracts from the adrenal cortex, work that would win him (with E. C. Kendall and Tadeus Reichstein) a well-deserved Nobel Prize. Among those extracts was a substance he called Compound E, which had a startling impact on rheumatoid arthritis. The compound soon became known throughout the world as cortisone.

Cortisone was among the most miraculous of the new wonder drugs that followed World War II. It was absolutely astonishing to see its effects on patients who had been bedridden with crippling, advanced rheumatoid arthritis: they were suddenly able to rise and walk again without pain.

Most of America's rheumatologists quickly decided that the natural cortisone production in the body of an arthritic patient was simply too low, much as natural insulin production is too low in the body of a diabetic. This concept of arthritis as a kind of deficiency replaced whatever was left of the infectious theory, and much of the medical world celebrated the conquest of the world's most prevalent disease—even though the deficiency thesis was unproven and the cause of the alleged deficiency was still undetermined.

In fact, I knew from my own research that the thesis was not only unproven, but its basic premise was incorrect. The question of the role played by the glands in arthritis—the adequacy of the thyroid, the ovaries, or the adrenal gland, or the other endocrines—had been investigated extensively. It was known that the adrenal gland, where cortisone is made, was no different in arthritic patients than in patients without any trace of arthritis.

Yet the paradox remained that an excessive level of cortisone—far above what was being produced normally—would make an arthritic patient feel better. Supporters of the deficiency theory amended their thesis slightly to fit the results: they decided that although arthritics did indeed produce a normal amount of cortisone in their own bodies, it was of an inferior quality. No evidence was ever given to show in what way it was inferior or that it differed in any way from the cortisone produced by people who were perfectly healthy.

On the contrary, new evidence soon appeared that placed the deficiency theory in even more serious doubt. With a true deficiency, as in hypothyroidism, for example, replacement of the missing endocrine permits the body to keep functioning indefinitely at its normal levels; patients who take daily doses of thyroid to supplement or replace the production of a damaged or missing thyroid gland lead otherwise normal lives. But with this new "cure" for arthritis, it became apparent that after a relatively short time, usually within just a few months, the extra cortisone began to lose its effectiveness.

PROBLEMS IN PARADISE

Hench's work and the results his compound at first achieved so captured the enthusiasm of the medical world that even when cortisone's effectiveness began to decline, almost nobody wanted to turn back from the new deficiency theory that its discovery had generated. Hench himself explained the failure as a problem of the kind of cortisone that was being used, and he exhorted the medical world to find a more effective type that would last indefinitely.

For the next decade, an enormous campaign of scientific research produced one steroid after another in the hope of finding such an ideal product. But after ten years of high promises followed by inevitably dismal disappointments, the great enthusiasm behind the quest for the perfect cortisone finally began to fizzle out.

A very big additional reason for the steroid fizzle was the discovery of numerous negative effects. These included stomach ulcers, high blood pressure, diabetes, and cataracts, among other things. It was observed that in many cases, prolonged and excessive use of cortisone resulted in the loss of calcium from the bones, a fact of particular concern to older patients already suffering from osteoporosis. If arthritis were really caused by a natural deficiency, we knew from our experience with hypothyroidism that the missing endocrine could be replaced for the rest of the patient's life and no such side effects would ever arise. Even with the eventual shift away from steroids, however, the deficiency concept tarried on.

When Hench suggested the problems with cortisone were just with its form, I finally began to object in public. I was certain that the adverse effects arose from the cortisone itself, and not just because the compound needed some fine tuning. I believed that cortisone's anti-inflammatory properties could still serve physicians who wanted to use the drug as an adjunct to some other form of treatment; indeed, I still use low levels to help patients through the initial stages of antibiotic therapy, or in cases where earlier misuse of steroids has destroyed the patient's ability to produce the required natural amount. But I was certain that the ways in which cortisone had been used for the ten years following its discovery had produced far more serious problems than the ones it had resolved. And I was also sure, as was the rest of the medical world by then, that whatever good things cortisone seemed to do at first, the benefits didn't last.

The impact of the discovery of cortisone on arthritis research was very similar to that of the discovery of insulin, in the early 1920s, on diabetes research. Both discoveries abruptly ended nearly all ongoing efforts to find the causes of their respective diseases. Nobody seemed to care what made arthritis or diabetes happen as long as they could control the symptoms. Years later, it was discovered that it wasn't enough just to manage blood-sugar levels with insulin, that the long-term complications from diabetes, such as retinal damage, cataracts, infections, and abscesses, still occurred.

THE ROMANCE COOLS

With the cortisone honeymoon approaching its end in the early 1960s, the American Rheumatism Association began to take a more prudent view of the use of steroids in large doses, but the medical community was still a long way from suing for divorce. Cortisone was still wonderful; it was just not as wonderful as it had been in 1950, and it had to be used in a more gingerly fashion. Although it was not said explicitly, there was a tacit recognition that what had been reluctantly identified as side effects of cortisone were not side effects at all; they were normal effects, part and parcel of using steroids in large quantities. And they could be disastrous.

Ironically, the effects of excessive cortisone had been identified and spelled out in detail a number of years earlier by the great neurosurgeon Harvey Cushing. Cushing's syndrome is a condition in which the pituitary gland, which is at the base of the brain, becomes overactive. When that happens, it makes the adrenal gland overactive as well, and the result is that the body produces too much cortisone. The effects Cushing noted from the overproduction of natural cortisone include hypertension, diabetes, cataracts, ulcers, osteoporosis, and odd distribution of body fat so that the torso becomes very large while the legs and arms remain small. Diabetes, mellitus, impotence in men, and hirsutism in women were also features of the clinical pattern. Cushing never called these phenomena side effects because he knew that they weren't side effects; they were the regular effects of too much cortisone. They had been an important part of the literature for decades.

For the whole field of arthritis research, there was a very costly long-term legacy from the introduction and spectacular early success of cortisone. That success was responsible for a nearly total commitment to the study and treatment of rheumatoid arthritis as a metabolic process, at the expense of any further study of the question of a primary infectious component. It was finally found that cortisone owed its effects to the fact that it interfered in some way with the autoimmune reaction, that it made people feel remarkably better almost immediately because it blocked the body's natural defenses. When it became apparent that the benefits didn't hold up over time, the medical profession found itself in the midst of a terrible dilemma. On one side was the immense early promise that had attached to a product that may well be the most highly publicized drug in the history of medicine. On the other was the growing body of evidence that it didn't last, and that the patient could wind up worse off than when the treatment started.

That pattern—enormous early promise, followed by terrible disillusionment—was to be repeated over and over again as an endless succession of new metabolic compounds flowed from the research laboratories of America and the rest of the world. Indeed, it would characterize the course of arthritis research for most of the next thirty years.

CORTISONE IS STILL USEFUL

I recognized that cortisone had some valuable properties in the treatment of arthritis, but from the very beginning I opposed the enthusiasm for large doses of any compound that would totally block the body's immune defense system. Cortisone in those quantities was being used like a dam in a river, and I knew that the pressure would continue to build and that sooner or later the dam would break or overflow—usually with a peptic ulcer that would start to bleed, so treatment had to be stopped—and the rebound flare would create disastrous consequences for the patient. And that is exactly what happened. When the use of cortisone at these high levels finally failed, most of the medical world had subscribed too heavily to the autoimmune theory to switch back to the possibility of infection playing a role.

Meanwhile, my own group continued working in the same old direction. Even when cortisone was at its peak of popularity, before the failures had mounted into the millions, we assumed that if there were an infectious allergy from mycoplasmas or anything else, cortisone worked simply because it blocked the allergy, not because it supplanted any natural deficiency or cured a thing. Cortisone's effect on allergies had already been well established; when people suffered from very severe status asthmaticus, for example, and were practically dead with breathing problems, cortisone would stop the attack right away by blocking the allergic reaction. Because rheumatoid arthritis responded so well, at first, to this anti-allergy substance, we began to speculate that the disease involved more of an allergic reaction than anyone had previously assumed, and we began to investigate that avenue as well. In regular allergies, the main offender is histamine release. In rheumatoid hypersensitivity, histamine is present in small amounts; the main offender is a mixture of proteolytic enzymes.

Despite its failures, over the course of the following years I frequently acknowledged our debt to cortisone for the redirection it had given to scientific thought on the question of hypersensitivity or the allergic state. It became well known that when a physician used cortisone in large quantities, and especially when that use led to dramatic remission, the disease got ten times worse when the cortisone was finally stopped. This backlash wasn't just a subjective observation of patients; it was detectable in the sudden increases in rheumatoid factor, sedimentation rate, gamma globulin, and reactive proteins, in the fall in hemoglobin, and in all the other measurable indicators by which the disease is monitored.

BACK TO THE DRAWING BOARD

Once the deficiency theory had finally run its course, the medical and scientific world slowly returned to an examination of some of the alternative causes of rheumatoid arthritis. The theory is now gradually reemerging that an infection or some other form of antigen creates a reaction which in turn causes inflammation in the joints, pain, weakness, and the other classic symptoms of the disease.

One of the first places medical researchers began to look after cortisone fizzled out was toward nonsteroidal anti-inflammatories. Suddenly a flood of such drugs appeared on the market: Naprosyn, Nalfon, Tolectin, Meclomen, Clinoril, and many more. They were designed to do what cortisone did in blocking inflammation, but without the side effects. All of these compounds passed the standard six-month double-blind screening requirements of the FDA, and they were all very promising. But over the course of longer experience, sometimes only after a couple of years of clinical use by hundreds of thousands of patients, many of the old, invidious side effects inevitably reemerged, along with some new ones. Some of these drugs caused stomach troubles; others have been discovered to cause kidney damage.

The primary impetus for the eventual turning away from cortisone, as indeed from all the other standard methods of symptomatic therapy, including gold and methotrexate in more recent years, has not been the doctors; it has been the patients. A lot of doctors resist the notion that there may be some democracy in medicine, and their resistance has slowed down the shift of arthritis research back toward treatments the patient can live with. The fact is that people are not going to tolerate medication that could easily destroy their health or their lives. Patients should be brought into the process of setting directions far sooner than they are, and they should be included deliberately, not just after everything has failed.

Most doctors pay lip service to the concept that patients should have some say in their treatment, but very few are really eager to see a system in which information about how medicines work is systematically shared and becomes the primary mechanism for setting the direction of treatment and research. A doctor feels that he is blessed with profound knowledge, as indeed he is. And he has been through the mill to learn what he knows: he's suffered through incredibly hard work in four years of college, four years of medical school, and four years of hospital training. As a rule, the patient has little of this breadth of knowledge. Patients often have a particular understanding of their own disease, however, which they have acquired from extensive reading and from conversations with others who suffer from the same affliction. The patient has something else which is extremely valuable and which many doctors do not have: direct experience with the failure or success of the various medicines which the doctor prescribes. That knowledge is absolutely imperative to the process by which such products are refined and future medicines are developed.

BREACH OF PROMISE

For most rheumatoid arthritics, this long history of broken promises and misdirections has been one of the most painful aspects of their disease. And it has created a reaction: the problem of false hope has emerged as one of the most important factors in gaining a consensus and setting the agenda for arthritis research. Patients who have been told that wonderful things will happen, only to discover that the effects don't last and that they often carry a terrible price, finally reach a point where they no longer believe in anything. That one problem, more than anything else, provides the best reason for directing research toward the cause of arthritis instead of toward its symptoms. Any medicine that eliminates the source of the problem cannot fail.

One of the things we have repeatedly demonstrated with our research on mycoplasmas is that when the treatment is aimed at the primary antigen that causes the arthritis reaction, a lot of the symptomatic drugs which had previously failed to be effective will come back to life again. An attack on the antigen itself even revives the efficacy of aspirin in patients for whom aspirin had stopped relieving pain many years earlier. Many new patients ask me what I can give them to supplant their most recent painkiller because, like all the others, it has stopped working. I tell them that I'll do something even better than that; I'll continue them on the old painkiller and make it work again.

WHY SYMPTOMATIC REMEDIES FAIL

The reason all such pain medicines eventually fail when the patient is treated symptomatically is not that the patient's system is getting any weaker, but that the antigen is becoming that much more widespread. When any such medicine removes the inflammatory barrier from around the source of the antigen, it is like removing the coolant from a nuclear power core, and the eventual result is a meltdown. The inflammation is nature's way of holding the reaction in check; it happens to be a painful method, but it is the only means by which the spread of the source of the antigen is contained. The fact that aspirin and other painkillers can be made to work again after the patient has started tetracycline therapy is more than a convenience for the management of discomfort. It is one further indication that the antibiotic is attacking the problem at its source.

LIKE A BACTERIAL ALLERGY

Essentially, rheumatoid arthritis operates in the manner of a bacterial allergy, leading to collagen vascular disturbances. It is an allergic or hypersensitive state. The reaction is most intense in the connective tissue between the cells.

By itself, each of these pieces of the rheumatoid arthritis puzzle may be little more than a curiosity. But taken together, a complete picture has formed over time, and it now provides researchers with their first full portrait of the process by which rheumatoid arthritis occurs. Only with this portrait in mind can a plan for sustained control and ultimate elimination of the disease be designed.

CHAPTER 14

Curly Knowlton

Some years ago, I had a patient named Curly Knowlton. He was a great outdoorsman, and such an expert fisherman that he could put a fly on a dime at a hundred feet—a skill which he had often demonstrated at Madison Square Garden, as well as along the banks of rivers and streams all through the American and Canadian Rockies. He supported this avocation by writing for fishing magazines and running an anglers' supply company. One day, he began to have trouble with his knees. He bought an exercise bicycle to help build them up to their old tone, but the treatment seemed to make his condition worse than before. By the time someone finally put him in touch with me, he was so badly crippled that he had been confined to a wheelchair for several months and was unable to take a step without help.

I was head of medicine at George Washington University at the time, and I recognized in Curly's situation a rare opportunity to make a dramatic point with our medical students. I learned early on that, in general, medical students don't have much interest in arthritis; they dismiss the victims as people who are simply worn out, and not worth the trouble.

And it isn't just doctors. In some respects, the unspoken

popular attitude toward arthritis seems to be that it is part of a sort of natural selection process in which nature culls out the weak. Rheumatoid arthritis afflicts three times as many women as men, is seldom fatal in its own right, and is a disease which is judged falsely as an affliction of unsturdy people whose fabric is basically flawed. Worse yet, most of the people who suffer from rheumatoid arthritis have a hang-dog attitude toward themselves and their affliction; acute depression is as real a part of the pathology as the pain and crippling. Arthritics have a hard time fighting back because they don't feel they really *deserve* much better—and that attitude may be the one contagious part of the disease.

The day the demonstration began, we collected a very large group of medical students, interns, residents, and nurses, and crowded them all into the patient's room. I knew Curly well enough to call him by his nickname at that point (he didn't have a hair on his head), and I offered him the following proposition. "Curly," I said, "I want you to cooperate in a procedure here that you may find very difficult. I'm going to ask you to stay in bed for as long as it takes us to cure your arthritis. Don't get up for anything—not even to go to the bathroom. I want to be sure that you don't give your legs any exercise at all. You've been working every day to try to make them better with your exercise bicycle, but now we're going in exactly the opposite direction and you won't do anything."

"Good God," Curly said, "if I don't have some kind of activity, I'll just fall apart!" He was a wonderful foil for my intended demonstration, and I could see that his protests were producing a dramatic effect on the audience.

"Well, I want to prove something, and this is the only way I know how," I said. "What I want to prove is that in two weeks' time, without doing a single thing yourself to improve your condition, you're going to get up out of that bed and walk all the way down the hall to the nurses' desk."

"Hell," Curly said, "that's just plain impossible." He looked to his audience, apparently hoping to find a reprieve from someone in the group who felt as strongly as he did that my plan would never work. Perhaps Curly didn't fully appreciate the relationship between a head of medicine and his students in a medical school; I, too, detected a good deal of sympathy for his position from the two dozen-odd faces around the crowded room, but no such reprieve was forthcoming—in fact, no one said a word.

"What I'm doing here is putting my reputation on the line," I told Curly and the students. "And I'm not about to make a wild claim that I can't live by. If you give me the two weeks, I'll put you back on your feet."

Realizing that he didn't have a single advocate in the roomful of sympathizers, Curly laid his head back on the pillow in defeat. Finally he looked warily back at me and asked, "How are you going to do it?" He didn't seem very interested in the answer.

"I'll treat you intravenously with an antibiotic. It will put out the fire of the disease activity in your knees or at least quiet it down, and reduce the toxins that are running up your legs and weakening your muscles. Your muscles will automatically be strengthened just by the absence of the destructive activity that's going on around them, and they will do that without exercise."

I wasn't taking any risk at all, either with my reputation or with Curly's health. If he promised not to get out of bed, I knew enough about his character to be sure he'd stick with it. And I had enough experience in treating rheumatoid arthritis to be certain of obtaining the promised results. I also knew that if I hoped to teach my students anything about how tetracycline works on arthritis, I would have to firmly close the door to any possible claim that Curly had simply exercised himself back to good health.

He waved a weak hand in affirmation. "Okay, you have a deal."

I told the medical students and the others in the audience to return there in exactly two weeks, and I named the time.

For the next fourteen days, Curly was treated with intravenous doses of tetracycline, and I checked on him and his nurses several times a day to verify that he was keeping his word about the exercise. I didn't doubt him, but I wanted to make sure that nobody missed the point.

We reassembled at the designated hour, and this time I realized that there were even more people in the room than had been there two weeks before, including some physicians from the hospital staff. I stood by the head of Curly's bed and in due course I asked him if he had followed our agreement and stayed in bed the whole time.

"Yes," he said, without much enthusiasm. "I didn't get up one single time."

"And did you take any form of exercise?"

"No," he said. "How could I?"

"All right," I said. "Now let me just ask you, Curly: Do you think that without treatment there are any circumstances under which you could have gotten out of this bed and walked down to the nurses' station?"

"No," he said, his voice rising with the anger and frustration that had been building up over the past fourteen days, "and by God I don't think there is any chance at all that I can do it now, either. I came here in a wheelchair because I couldn't walk in the first place, and I've been lying here flat on my back ever since, going to seed."

"Well," I said, "try it and we'll have a chance to see."

I pulled back the covers from his bed. He swung his legs over the side and, after a moment's hesitation, stood up. One of the nurses reached out to take his arm, but I motioned for her to step aside. Some of the spectators who crowded around the doorway backed out into the corridor as Curly put one shaky leg in front of the other and started unsteadily across the room. No one in the entire company looked more astonished than Curly himself. He rounded the corner into the hallway, and a few moments later he stood triumphantly in front of the nurses' station. Then he executed a smart about-face and walked with increasing confidence and delight back to where the grand procession had begun.

Curly's arthritis was on the mend. More to the point, from

that day forward there was a whole new generation of students at George Washington University School of Medicine who decided that arthritis was worth treating after all, that there may very well be a cause that can be defined, and that there was a treatment that could actually work.

CHAPTER 15

The Case Against Double-Blind Testing

One of the most enduring and contentious impediments to the conquest of rheumatoid arthritis has been the lack of an effective methodology to test its various forms of treatment. What drugs work, how do they work, and for how long do they work? What are their good effects and what are their bad ones?

There are now some two thousand remedies for arthritis. Some of them are old wives' tales, some are herbs or other natural products, and many hundreds of them are the results of pharmaceutical research based on the premise that the disease is a metabolic disorder of unknown cause. The standard medicines that have already been used on a typical arthritic before I take the case represent the best and most popular of this last class of treatment. Every one of them has passed the standard six-month double-blind crossover tests used for judging pharmaceutical compounds, and every one of them is ineffective in controlling the progress of the disease.

Double-blind testing is the method in which neither the doctor nor the patient knows whether the substance being administered is a true medicine or a placebo that does nothing. The test group is divided equally, and only when the six-month trial period has elapsed is it revealed which half got the real thing. Meanwhile, each patient's progress is followed closely for reactions and for diagnostic indications of improvement or decline.

WHY THE DOUBLE-BLIND STANDARD?

The reason this method has been successful in the development of many other kinds of medicine is that the process is beyond partisan control, and the results are free of interpretive bias. Double-blind testing works just fine when the response is linear and the process being examined is completed within the six-month test period.

The reason it does not work with drugs used in the treatment of rheumatoid arthritis is that the response is not linear and the process by which the body reacts to the medicine is seldom completed within six months. The indications of how well the drug is working can reverse themselves shortly after the product has been certified as safe, and overnight the beneficial medicine can become a deadly poison. Of all the hundreds of metabolic or symptomatic drugs that have been developed against rheumatoid arthritis over the past four decades, not a single one has stayed effective and nontoxic for a period of five years. And it is not uncommon for patients who have taken part in a double-blind study to admit that they did not adhere to the rules—that they took other medicine when the pain became too intense.

TOO LITTLE DATA, TOO LATE

Double-blind testing doesn't work with antibiotic therapy for essentially the same reason, but with exactly the opposite result: in cases of deeply entrenched rheumatoid arthritis, six months isn't long enough for the treatment to produce a beneficial effect—indeed, because of the Herxheimer reaction, during the test period the patient's condition can actually get worse.

That dual paradox is the essential flaw of the double-blind approach: the drugs that look good in the short term ultimately prove to be worse than worthless; the only medications that produce lasting benefits are the ones which six-month double-blind testing would be likely to eliminate at the start. In fact, one of the reasons for the failure of the so-called Boston Study of a few years ago, in which the effects of tetracycline therapy were analyzed in seventeen rheumatoid arthritics, was that it stopped too soon. (There were several other reasons: the low number of cases, the wrong frequency in administration of the antibiotic; and the fact that more than half the patients were receiving other medications at the same time.)

ALTERNATIVES

Recently a doctor in the Infectious Disease Institute of the National Institutes of Health isolated a strain of mycoplasma from the joint fluid of a human with rheumatoid arthritis. Such isolations are no longer unusual and several others, including ourselves, have done the same thing. What was unusual was that the NIH doctor then inoculated a chimpanzee with this human strain of mycoplasma and induced arthritis in the animal. This animal model provides the perfect opportunity to prove cause and effect and to provide a means for controlling drug testing.

It would be far better to return to the method we used in the past: evaluating a drug over a five-year period, and comparing this with data already accumulated on the effect of gold for the same period of time. Such a comparison has been made with data supplied from our Arthritis Institute. Ninety-nine patients who had been treated with the antibiotic approach over a five-year period were selected for this study. Most of these patients had previously discontinued standard remedies, because they became toxic or ineffective. The data were examined by an independent statistical group who agreed that our results were valid. A comparison was made with the published data on a hundred patients who were treated with gold for a period of five years. More than 80 percent of our patients who had been treated with antibiotics were still improving after five years, whereas only 10 percent of the patients treated with gold were still on the drug. The other 90 percent of the gold patients had dropped out for the familiar reason: the gold had either become toxic or had lost its effectiveness.

In the case of AIDS research, there has been bitter, protracted debate regarding the need or justification for double-blind controls, and such controls are now no longer required in evaluating therapeutic results. A method of testing arthritis drugs that proceeds in the same manner as testing for AIDS medications would compare the failures and successes of different compounds in the same patients, not just for six months but for five years. This empirical approach would produce test information that is more relevant, far safer, and much more reliable than the double-blind method. It would not only reveal drugs that work, but exclude drugs that provide false hope—which in the long run only worsens the disease by increasing the stress from uncertainty and failure.

THE PRICE

The search for new, nonsteroidal anti-inflammatory drugs without toxic side effects and with the same pain-relieving qualities as cortisone has been enormously expensive, and the cost of the research has to be included in the retail price of the drugs. Many of the new compounds used for the treatment of arthritis were found to be toxic after they gained approval through six-month double-blind tests—and some of these delayed reactions proved to be lethal. Gold has been found to cause kidney trouble, and the newest form, oral gold, has been shown to suppress the formation of platelets and cause uncontrollable bleeding. Plaquenil has caused retinal damage, and penicillamine, which seemed to be remarkably effective when first used, has caused suppression of bone marrow in some people—and some deaths. The immunosuppressive drugs, such as methotrexate, have been found to damage the liver and sometimes the lungs.

Such complications have required intense monitoring of these drugs by the rheumatologist, ophthalmologist, and other specialists, all at considerable expense to the patient. Add the price of the drugs themselves, frequent laboratory tests, and costly treatments of the complications when they do occur, and a new perspective emerges on arthritis: its total cost to America is becoming far greater than that of the whole Vietnam War.

Fortunately, the risks associated with the standard treatments for arthritis are beginning to gain recognition at last and the circle is coming around again to a basic approach to the disease process. Medicine is getting back to where it was in the early 1950s, before the cortisone revolution. We are now standing at a crucial intersection in the quest for safety and security for the arthritic. We must continue in the right direction, focusing on the infectious concept with vigor, determination, and open-mindedness, qualities notably lacking in the past thirty years. Of the several hundred grants that have been made for arthritis research, less than a dozen have funded programs to probe the infectious theory.

One factor which has played a major role in the reversal of this inequity has been the appearance of Lyme disease.

CHAPTER 16

Lyme Disease: A Portrait of Infectious Arthritis

The formula for any good story is that it must have a beginning, a middle, and a conclusion, and at present Lyme disease is the form of arthritis that comes closest to meeting that requirement; the model it provides for future researchers should eventually lead to a full library of happy endings. For most people, including lovers of detective stories and romantics who like to see everything properly disposed of and explained in the end, the story of Lyme disease is a classic thriller. For diehard advocates of the metabolic theory of rheumatoid arthritis, however, the final chapter brings some very unsettling news.

The first reported cases of Lyme disease were in 1975, in the town on the eastern shore of the Connecticut River that gives the affliction its name. Two mothers called the state health department to say that their children had just been diagnosed as having rheumatoid arthritis, and they suspected an epidemic. Juvenile rheumatoid arthritis can be a very serious disease, and when the department looked into the situation they found that indeed there were several other cases in the vicinity, as well an inordinate number of adult cases reported in the same period.

The health authorities called Yale University School of Medicine and spoke with a postdoctoral fellow in rheumatology named Allen Steere. Steere took on the puzzle. He started by calculating that the thirty-nine children and twelve adult cases diagnosed to that date represented a rate of incidence a hundred times higher than normal for the size of the population. Moreover, in areas where cases of the disease clustered—heavily wooded rural sites—the rate was ten thousand times higher than it should have been.

Steere then identified several important features of the epidemic. From the pattern of dates on which families and neighbors showed their first symptoms, he concluded that it was a summertime affliction and that it was not highly contagious, which is to say that those afflicted were not catching it from one another but from some other source. A clue to that unknown source was found in the fact that a quarter of the victims recalled having an unusual rash a couple of days to a month before the first signs of arthritis, and the distribution and form of the rash suggested the bite of a crawling insect or spider.

PATTERN RECOGNITION

Steere also discovered that the same skin rash pattern had been reported in Europe in 1909, although without the subsequent arthritis, and that it had been traced to the bite of a tick, *Ixodes ricinus*. Some decades later, cases of that same rash pattern in Europe were treated with penicillin and cured, from which scientists inferred that the active agent in 1909 had been a bacterial infection. Accordingly, an attempt was made to isolate bacteria from the synovial fluid of several victims of the Lyme epidemic, but nothing showed up.

A couple of years after he started, Steere had a piece of extraordinary luck: one of the people who came down with the disease in 1977 not only recalled having been bitten by a tick—but he had saved it. Steere sent the tick up to Harvard, where it was identified as *Ixodes dammini*, a close cousin of the

European protagonist of seventy years earlier. Distribution studies subsequently established *Ixodes dammini* as the likely vector, or carrier, of Lyme disease.

SPIROCHETE INFECTION

That still didn't explain what Lyme disease was. Many ticks were gathered from the wild, but studies of their organs and digestive systems were no more productive than the earlier work with human joint fluid. Four years later, however, other scientists researching an outbreak of Rocky Mountain spotted fever opened the digestive system of an *Ixodes dammini* and found that it was filled with spirochete bacteria. They knew that the tick was the prime suspect in Lyme disease, and they guessed that the spirochete was the long-sought infectious agent. Subsequently the connection was proven. DNA studies showed the spirochete was a new species, which was named *Borrelia burgdorferi* after the researcher who first saw it.

Researchers who studied Lyme disease under a grant from the National Institutes of Health have identified three clinical stages, although not all patients demonstrate all stages. The first, showing up within a few days to a month after the bite, can include migratory rash, fatigue, fever, chills, and aches. The second stage can include irregular electrical activity in the heart muscle, showing up as shortness of breath, dizziness, and palpitations. The third stage is arthritis, sometimes accompanied by disorientation and memory loss. All three of those stages can vary widely, and Lyme disease is frequently misdiagnosed, often as Alzheimer's or multiple sclerosis.

KNOCKING IT OUT

Even if treatment waits until the third stage, either penicillin or tetracycline is still effective in knocking out most cases, although the NIH-sponsored researchers found that some entrenched incidents require that the antibiotics be administered intravenously. They also noted that several physicians treating the arthritic stage of the disease had encountered the Herxheimer effect, in which the symptoms became temporarily worse once treatment began, and they suspected that this reaction was another important clue. Subsequent laboratory tests showed that the Herxheimer effect probably results from the release of powerful agents from the walls of the dying bacteria as they are attacked by the antibiotic; these, in turn, stimulate the host body's immune defense mechanism.

That same chain reaction accounts for the Herxheimer effect in every other rheumatoid form of arthritis, whether the invading agent is a spirochete, streptococcus, or mycoplasma.

Of course, the chain reaction of rheumatoid arthritis doesn't begin or end with the Herxheimer effect. In the more common forms of arthritis, for example, we have known for a long time that mycoplasmas localize, and that if you can get them out of the joints, in most cases the condition will improve. We also know, even accounting for the Herxheimer effect, that if we're progressing at a good rate and the patient is getting better, it very often happens that some other bacterial antigen will enter the picture and make matters worse again. What has occurred in those instances is that the antigens from the mycoplasma or some other disease agent have sensitized the area in question, so that future incidents now have an easy place to happen.

When the stage is set in that way, lots of other factors can get into the act. Medication and foods can become serious problems, for example, as the sensitized body begins to reject them. Sinus troubles or kidney problems can appear. Antigens of many different types can enter the picture and create chaos.

SLEEPER

One of the sleeping antigens that is very hard to measure is streptococcus. It has been well established that the toxins from streptococci, as well as those from mycoplasmas, have an affinity for joints. We have found in the course of taking comprehensive histories of our patients that a tremendous number of them have had severe troubles with their sinuses or their tonsils or their ears, or have had scarlet fever or rheumatic fever—all streptococcal conditions. Strep is an organism that is very susceptible to penicillin, which is why rheumatic fever and scarlet fever are no longer the terrible menaces they were a generation ago. But even after it has been knocked out as a source of infection, streptococcus hangs on for years—in tonsils, around teeth, and in other hiding places—not causing infection, but serving as another source of antigen, or toxin, with that demonstrated specificity for joints.

In treating rheumatoid arthritis, when a physician gets to the point with tetracycline therapy that the mycoplasmas have been substantially reduced and further progress appears to be limited, it makes sense to probe the possibility that streptococcus is complicating the process. If a titer of streptococcal antibodies indicates that their levels are elevated, then both the mycoplasma and the strep can be treated at the same time, continuing tetracycline for the former and using ampicillin for the latter.

Nothing about rheumatoid arthritis is simple, and it doesn't necessarily stop there; the streptococcus often alters its form (see discussion of L-form in Chapter 18), which further compounds the problem. Treatment of the strep then takes one kind of medication, and treatment of the altered form requires yet another.

THE INFECTIOUS ALLERGY

All of these scenarios follow the pattern of infectious allergies, which is one of the central processes of all forms of rheumatoid arthritis and which must be addressed in their treatment. Lyme disease is harder to cure the longer it remains untreated; when the allergic reaction has been given enough time to become securely established, the resistance to therapy can be multiplied many times over. The same applies to all other forms of rheumatoid arthritis.

Finally, for those who like a moral with their short stories, it should be acknowledged that Lyme disease proves once again that there is no such thing as a panacea in dealing with mankind's oldest disease. Tetracycline may be all a doctor could ask for in treating many other forms of rheumatoid arthritis—even most of them—but by itself it is still not the whole answer.

The whole answer is in the one area that has received the least attention in the past forty years and that has finally been illuminated by the brilliant research which solved the puzzle of Lyme disease: a complete understanding of the causes of rheumatoid arthritis and of the mechanism by which it occurs.

CHAPTER 17

Tomoka: The First Animal Model

Tomoka is a silver-back gorilla, and he lives at the National Zoo in Washington, D.C. Twenty-six years ago, Tomoka made headlines as the second gorilla ever to be born in captivity in the United States, the fourth such captive birth in the world.

Despite the national attention he received by virtue of his origins, Tomoka is a perfect example of the fickleness of fame; by the time he was five years old, most of his adoring public had abandoned him and he was a has-been. His growth had stopped at a frail 150 pounds, and he sat in the corner of his cage rubbing his joints and looking miserable. A terribly sick gorilla in the zoo represents the same kind of liability as a waiting room full of sick, depressed humans in a doctor's office—it is a downer, and reflects poorly on those in charge. Nobody likes to spend his free time witnessing that kind of embarrassment. In addition, the animal was suffering from a great deal of pain and had not responded to more than twenty different remedies used for the treatment of arthritis in humans.

We were called by zoo officials and asked if we would be interested in having pathological material to study when they put him to sleep, which was planned to be carried out in a few days. We asked to see Tomoka, examine him, and do studies of his blood before they carried out their plans, and they agreed.

It soon became clear that we were seeing the first model of human rheumatoid arthritis ever encountered in an animal. Our success in treating humans with the antibiotic approach was well known in the Washington community, and with some persuasion the zoo officials allowed us to treat the gorilla with intravenous tetracycline; we in turn agreed that if there was no response, then they should carry out their plans. I did point out that it might take some time before Tomoka showed signs of improvement, and they agreed to accept this arrangement.

Tomoka was treated with intravenous tetracycline by drip every two weeks. Although he got worse at the outset of therapy, he gradually began to get better, gaining in strength and then in weight. We have now followed Tomoka for more than twenty years. His flare reactions progressively lessened in both frequency and intensity over approximately a three-year period, and he has remained completely well for the balance of that time. He is now a healthy, strong, very active, full-grown gorilla. He has only one toe that bears the remains of some cartilaginous destruction, and that in no way hinders his activity.

Since Tomoka's case was reported, we have been in touch with a great many zoos which have told us of similar cases. We have advised our treatment, and there are now more than thirty gorillas that we know of that are doing well under this program. We also know of two gorillas that were treated by standard methods and died; we are not sure of the cause of death.

Dr. Dan Laughlin, a veterinarian at the Chicago Zoo, told me of the zoo's success in treating one of their gorillas who had arthritis similar to Tomoka's. Dr. Laughlin came to see me because of his own arthritis and I learned that he had seen a great deal of arthritis in elephants, which was his area of special interest. Dr. Harold Clark, our research associate, has pursued laboratory studies of the elephants and a number of strains of mycoplasma comparable to those in the gorillas have been detected by mycoplasma complement fixing reactions in the blood.

Tomoka's care and the results of his treatment have attracted a lot of attention as well as controversy, although among veterinarians there is only enthusiasm. An article in the *Washington Post* in April 1984 says of these veterinarians, "They are . . . convinced that Brown's treatment . . . has essentially eliminated rheumatoid arthritis as a major threat to zoos and circuses."

CHAPTER 18

How Arthritis Happens: The Mechanism

The idea that there is a viruslike agent or some kind of invisible infectious component in the tissues affected by arthritis had its start in work done at the Rockefeller Institute between 1936 and 1939. The results of that work were published first in a brief article in *Science* in 1939, and then elaborated some ten years later in the rheumatic disease section of *Post Graduate Medicine and Surgery*. A paper by Dr. Louis Dienes and Howard Weinberger entitled "Experimental Arthritis: Pleuropneumonia-like Organisms and their Possible Relation to Articular Disease" spoke of the L-form of bacteria as "an invisible, filterable form that may exist after the parent germ disappears."

THE L-FORM

I had arrived at a similar understanding through my own observations in the late 1930s, but from a different point of view. I had gone to the Rockefeller Institute to try to disclose the presence of some virus or infection in rheumatic tissues, using embryonated hen's eggs as the tissue on which to grow the organisms. All of my results had been negative for the first three or four months; I had inoculated hundreds of eggs, and nothing at all had shown up on the membrane. Finally, when something did appear, it turned out to be the so-called L-form, or what we thought was bacteria. (The L-form took its name from the Lister Institute in London, where it was first described by Dr. Emmy Klieneberger. It was not until some years later that a committee of the American Microbiological Society decided to give this class of organisms a more formidable name. *Mycoplasma* derives from the Latin base words for fungus and fluid.)

By isolating a strain of the L-form organism from a Bartholin cyst, which occurs on female labia, Dienes became the first researcher to observe it in humans. I was the first one to find an L-form strain in joints and to connect it to arthritis.

WHY THINGS SOMETIMES GET WORSE BEFORE THEY GET BETTER

I was asked to write a discussion of the Dienes-Weinberger paper, and I reported that we had observed this organism in a number of clinical situations. Seventeen patients, representing a wide variety of rheumatic diseases including rheumatic arthritis, rheumatoid spondylitis, chorea, erythema nodosum, and rheumatic fever, were treated with Aureomycin, a tetracycline derivative, because it had an effect on these organisms. As an interesting corollary, we noted that gold salts produced approximately the same result. And we were also impressed that when we started treating these patients with a tetracycline product (the Aureomycin), they invariably got worse before they started getting better—a phenomenon in medicine known as the Jarisch-Herxheimer reaction.

This discussion was the first linking in the entire medical literature of the Jarisch-Herxheimer effect with a tetracycline derivative in a rheumatic problem. Presumably the effect was due to the dislodging and breaking up of the mycoplasma and the releasing of antigen to a sensitized field. The effect showed a number of important principles at work. It demonstrated that the disease was a hypersensitive reaction, not to the drug itself but to the toxins that a germ creates in response to the drug's presence. It showed that the germ must indeed be invisible, as Dienes and Weinberger had suggested, because no other germs of such standard types as streptococcus and staphylococcus were isolable. And it opened the way to a chemical attack on the whole area of arthritis and rheumatic diseases.

HARD TO DO, HARD TO DUPLICATE

After our original research results were published in *Science* in 1939, our observations quickly became news. The *New York Times* ran a full page on the subject, and there was a lot of excitement among the media. But after a very short time, the excitement died.

The problem was that no one else was able to duplicate our results. This was thoroughly predictable; after all, it had taken me three months before I had been able to achieve those results in the first place, and other researchers tried it once or twice and gave up. When I left the Rockefeller Institute in 1939 and went back to Johns Hopkins to become chief resident in medicine, the school gave me a laboratory and eventually a fellow to pursue the subject further. I remained convinced that the subject was worth more work, but I found myself in a fast-shrinking minority in my conviction.

These original observations gave us a basis for looking at the possibility that rheumatoid arthritis was due to a kind of infectious allergy, and that mycoplasmas, unlike other germs that worked by invading the host, operated instead by sitting still in one place and giving off, in a pulsating fashion, something to which the body reacted. Because those emissions were irregular, there were periods when the disease was thoroughly quiescent and the person with arthritis would feel reasonably healthy. Conversely, there were other times—often associated with periods when the patient worked too hard or was under great stress or suffered an injury—when the hidden organism released toxins and the disease would flare up.

BREAKING THE EGG

It was one thing to infer the presence of mycoplasmas by observing their effects, but it was often quite another to study them at first hand. To begin with, they proved to be both extremely fragile and very good at hiding, not only on the host cell but within it. And if the research effort did anything to damage the area in which these tiny organisms were located, the mycoplasmas would quickly break up. When that happened, it was similar to an egg breaking in the refrigerator, with the remnants running everywhere.

Over the years, we studied what happens when the mycoplasmic egg is broken. We learned, eventually, that the toxin leaving the organism is not, in itself, particularly vicious; if it were, we realized that it would make the patient terribly sick, since a little bit of the toxin is escaping from the mycoplasma all the time. Instead, we came to understand that when the toxin is released over a period of months or years, it creates a reception by "fixed tissue antibodies" that are ready to react to these toxins every time they appear.

The way in which the body becomes sensitized to mycoplasmas is similar to the way in which it learns to react to poison ivy. First-time visitors to the United States could take a shower in poison ivy resins, and the only thing most of them would get from it would be sticky. Until the body produces an antibody or allergen, there's no reaction. By the same token, one could expect that it would take prolonged exposure to mycoplasma toxins before the stage would be properly set for a reaction to occur. Many of us could be carrying mycoplasmas from childhood—from an old infection, perhaps from viral pneumonia—that are ticking away inside our bodies, just waiting for that process to play itself out.

We also learned early on that mycoplasmas have a unique affinity for certain parts of the body, and they attach themselves there like no other germ. Most of what we know in that respect comes from work performed by other scientists on animals such as swine, chickens, and turkeys, particularly the research conducted by Albert Sabin on laboratory mice in which mycoplasmas were isolated, injected into the animals' bloodstreams, and headed unfailingly to the joints.

MYCOPLASMAS AND JOINTS

The history of science is filled with stories of major discoveries which seem so obvious in retrospect that one marvels at how long they remained unknown. The development of penicillin in 1928, for example, was greeted with universal delight, followed almost immediately by chagrin among several generations of physicians who, like Alexander Fleming, had observed the effects of mold on cultures growing in a petri dish but unlike him had inferred nothing useful from what they saw.

It is a lot easier to recognize a cure than to understand the mechanism of a disease, especially when the disease is as complex as rheumatoid arthritis. That principle may help us to understand why some of the most elemental properties of arthritis went unrecognized for decades after they should have become perfectly obvious. And it may help as well in explaining why arthritis has such a sorry history of "cures," many of which have proven more destructive than the disease itself.

The affinity of mycoplasmas for the tissue and fluid of the joints is just one such uniform factor that no one seemed to have noticed before, despite ample opportunities going back at least to the 1890s. At that time, a devastating epidemic of arthritis and pneumonia, called pleuropneumonia bovis, swept through the cattle herds of Europe, causing incredible mortality and raging across to the eastern end of Siberia. It was caused by a germ called *Streptobacillis moniliformis*, which grows in great chains in the culture media—and produces L-forms that mimic mycoplasmas. Scientists cultured the larger germ and, at a hundred magnifications on a microscope stage, they observed colonies of what looked like dozens and even hundreds of tiny fried eggs, unquestionably satellites to the parent organism. While they recognized that the satellite derived from the host, much as the moon originated in the area of the earth now occupied by the Pacific Ocean, they failed to understand that the fried eggs were another form of the same lethal agent and were at least as potent as the long strands of ropelike streptobacilli.

The satellite concept is useful in another way in appreciating how the mechanism of arthritis has remained so elusive. Let's suppose that a visitor from Mars were to visit the moon and ask the moon where it came from. If the moon could point to the earth and say, "I came from there," the Martian visitor shouldn't have much difficulty with that answer. But now suppose that something cataclysmic had happened after the moon was formed, and the earth was no longer there. It becomes a lot harder for the visitor to say, "I see," when the thing that he might have seen has disappeared.

THE GREAT DEBATE

This phenomenon of a kind of metamorphosis or variation from the streptobacillus into the L-form or mycoplasma—coupled with the disappearance of the original form—led to a tremendous debate between Dienes in the United States and Klieneberger in London. Dienes said that the mycoplasma derived from the streptobacillus with which it was originally intermingled and was another phase of the same creature. Klieneberger said the two phases were separate organisms, much as a pony is separate from a horse. The argument took on the aspects of a theological debate, Klieneberger representing the redoubtable Lister Institute, where the L-form had first been identified and after which it was named, and Dienes, on the other side of the ocean, releasing his arrows from behind the mighty ramparts of Harvard University.

Unhappily, as this battle raged, I found myself somewhere near the metaphoric equivalent of Bermuda, right in the middle. In my work at Johns Hopkins, we had recently isolated some streptobacillus from the joint fluid of a man who had been bitten by a rat. Streptobacillus was known to be carried by rats, and I recognized that the outcome of the debate would have profound implications for my work, and possibly vice versa.

In due course, Jack Nunemaker joined me and we were able to demonstrate that the L-form was a variant of the original streptobacillus organism, and we had reason to believe that all bacteria could indeed go into separate invisible forms. We showed that a germ could enter a state in which it could become invisible, pass through a filter, and then return to the parent form. It was a whole new world of subclinical phenomena, a world in which things could appear and disappear, take new shapes, be at once different and the same—the biochemical equivalent of solid ice changing into water or steam and back again as circumstances require. Was it possible, from the long persistence of the forms in tissues, that bacterial allergy would evolve?

ENTER, THE SHADOW

This view changed the way we looked at certain kinds of disease. A person could have osteomyelitis, for example, and the staphylococcus that caused it could clear up, leaving the patient fully healed, with no sign of the infectious agent no matter how many times it was cultured. But if that person then were to be given a lot of cortisone—enough to interfere with his immune mechanism—all of a sudden the old staphylococcus would come back to life again with a vengeance, returning to the visible world from out of nowhere, from out of the persisting invisible L-form.

When one accepts that Lamont Cranston is also the Shadow and can move back and forth between at least two states and maybe among several, it is easy to see implications for our understanding the mechanism of other diseases than arthritis. Multiple sclerosis, for example, and amyotrophic lateral sclerosis (Lou Gehrig's disease) have all kinds of invisible but seemingly infectious states.

From that point on, we continued looking for the L-form, or mycoplasma, separate from any other organism. I realized that we couldn't do this by inoculating tissues of animals or tissue cultures, because that procedure would leave us open to the suspicion of contamination. So instead we worked with exudates from the body and the blood directly into culture media, without using animals, eliminating the risk that we would pick up anything along the way. For thirty years, we tried to grow mycoplasmas from joint fluid, knowing from the start that they are extremely fragile structures and very difficult to cultivate outside the body.

LEARNING ABOUT MYCOPLASMA

Mycoplasmas are not viruses. True viruses require living cells in which to grow. Mycoplasmas are somewhere between a virus and a bacterium, but the real difference is that they contain RNA and DNA and are self-contained, living units. That difference is important, but their similarities to some viral forms were to prove instructive as well, especially when we began looking for mycoplasmas inside the human body and within living cells. A couple of years ago, armed with new, state-of-the-art equipment for electron microscopy and protein fractionation, we set about doing just that.

We were also armed with a formidable new director of research. Millicent Coker-Vann, with a Ph.D. in biochemistry in viral immunology, came to the Arthritis Institute from the National Institutes of Health, where she had been working in particular with the slow virus group. Although she had been connected with the NIH for more than a decade, along the way she taught for two years at the University of Ife in Nigeria, spent seven months as a fellow at the Max Planck Institute in West Germany, and received a research grant from the Rockefeller Foundation.

Breaking down the proteins of the body is somewhat like unwrapping a cocoon. Under Dr. Coker-Vann's guidance, we soon found that by fractionating the protein, we could easily layer off the mycoplasma antigen fraction, draw it off, put it in a rabbit, and develop antibodies against it which would match those of the patient. In a very short time, we were able to complete the circle back to the patient without having to isolate any of the elements from animal intermediaries.

Now we had both the mycoplasma antigen and the antibody in relation to the disease. We have found higher concentrations of both the antigen and the antibody in the joint fluid than in the blood. And the levels of both antigen and antibody have been noted to decrease following intravenous antimycoplasma therapy.

Early in the course of pursuing the new fractionation technology, we found that it wasn't necessary to have the whole living mycoplasmic organism to provoke the reaction in a joint or tissue. Our studies proved what we had previously been able to assume only by inference—that just the fragments of mycoplasmas were sufficiently potent to create a powerful antigenic reaction, causing the host to produce antibodies in reaction to their presence.

THE EVIDENCE ACCUMULATES

Over the course of time, we accumulated a larger and larger body of evidence that mycoplasmas were indeed the mechanism for rheumatoid arthritis.

First of all, only antimycoplasma drugs had any impact on

rheumatoid disease, except in those instances where there was a strong streptococcal connection. Ampicillin may be needed to lower the streptococcal antigen level and reduce symptoms. Tetracyclines were the only group of antibiotics we could find that suppress mycoplasma growth in the laboratory, and they were the only ones that seemed to improve the arthritis patients' conditions—unless there were other bacterial complications which added to the sensitizing process.

A further body of data was derived from studies of the other medicines, potions, and old wives' cures that have been used over the years to combat arthritis. Quinine is a long-time remedy for arthritis and a ubiquitous component of patent medicines that goes back centuries; it was used by our great-grandparents for backaches and rheumatism—so much so that many of our ancestors developed serious quinine allergies. We demonstrated, not surprisingly, that quinine has a specific effect on mycoplasmas, as does Plaquenil (hydroxychloroquine sulfate), another antimalarial substance to which quinine is closely related. Gold has also been found effective in suppressing mycoplasma growth, explaining its effectiveness in arthritis. We demonstrated the antimycoplasmic action of gold nearly forty years ago. Copper salts were first used by J. Forestier at about the same time he discovered the value of gold in rheumatoid disease, and he particularly noted their beneficial effect on rheumatoid arthritis; again, we demonstrated the ability of this substance to suppress mycoplasma growth. By the same token, it has been observed that copper bracelets react with perspiration to form copper salts, and work in Australia recently proved that those copper salts can penetrate the skin, which would explain the popularity of this preventive talisman from as long ago as the time of the ancient Romans.

Collectively, our observations confirmed a pattern in which mycoplasma could be seen as the consistent offender in the process by which rheumatoid arthritis occurs, and that pattern more than justified our efforts to isolate it.

We are also trying to "tag" the mycoplasma organism so we can see where it combines with human tissue. Tagging is a procedure by which the element under study is labeled with a tracer which signals its presence in microscopy. The reason for this approach is that without tagging, once the mycoplasma enters tissue, it is lost to view and can't be identified with any certainty, even with the electron microscope.

POINTING TO THE CAUSE OF RHEUMATOID ARTHRITIS

Regardless of what we learn about the final pieces of the rheumatoid arthritis puzzle in the time just ahead, I believe we already know enough about the mechanism—inferentially and from direct observation in our laboratory research, and from forty years of clinical experience—to state with certainty that mycoplasmas are the primary infectious agent, and that tetracycline therapy is the only effective therapy to reach toward the cure of rheumatoid arthritis.

The cause of rheumatoid arthritis is an antigenic substance which operates not as an invader, in the way of germs, but as the trigger for an internal allergic response, releasing toxins intermittently to a sensitized area, subsiding then reappearing We know that antibodies are transported throughout the body by white blood cells and platelets, much as smoke jumpers are carried by an airplane from one brush fire to the next. It is by this means that arthritis migrates, in the knee one day and in the shoulder or the back the next: the antigen builds up in the shoulder, and the antibody that was busy counteracting it in the knee moves on to the new battlefield, leaving the knee to a brief season of peace.

DEFLATING SOME MYTHS

Consider the alternatives. If one is to believe that rheumatoid arthritis is just a hereditary problem, or that it is due to stress or nutritional deficits or aging or a deficiency in the body's natural supply of cortisone, how is it possible to explain, for example, that the condition flares up the day before a storm comes?

One way in which myths are preserved is by the denial of evidence that would disprove them. Advocates of the genetic, nutritional, stress, aging, and cortisone-deficiency schools of arthritis simply dismiss the indications that arthritis is barometrically poised by calling them old wives' tales. But Dr. Joseph Hollander, the head rheumatologist at the University of Pennsylvania in Philadelphia, did a study some years ago of the effects on rheumatoid disease of barometric pressure, along with such other factors as temperature, humidity, and oxygen. He got volunteers to stay in sealed, climatically controlled rooms, writing their impressions of how they felt from hour to hour as he worked various subtle changes in their environment. It can be assumed that some of the changes, such as in humidity, might have been detectable through normal sensory means, but most of the changes were not. Hollander concluded, on the basis of excellent clinical evidence, that environment does indeed make a measurable difference in one's sensitivity to rheumatic disorders. Two factors were found to cause flare-ups: a sudden drop in barometric pressure, and the presence of high humidity in conjunction with such a drop. Both of them are common atmospheric characteristics prior to a storm. The barometric effect fits our concept perfectly by promoting a sudden release of antigen to a sensitized area.

I have always asked new patients about their experience with changes in weather, and also about their sensitivity to changes in the seasons. It has been well known for many years that patients with rheumatoid arthritis experience a higher incidence of flare-ups in the late spring and early fall. Very little work has been done in understanding the impact of seasonal changes on disease, although the increased incidence of depression that comes with the arrival of fall has been widely noted for a number of years, perhaps because it is supported by a measurable indicator in the form of a corresponding rise in the suicide rate. Our clinical experience with rheumatoid arthritis has shown that it, too, is subject to seasonality.

One other old wives' tale is worth examining for the clues it might provide to the arthritis mechanism, and that is the ancient belief that the pain in arthritic joints can be relieved by bee venom. This rather painful therapy is commonly practiced by the residents of New Hampshire, as indeed it is by rural folk throughout the world. New Hampshire happens to be favored by its proximity to Boston, and many members of the immense medical community in that city spend their weekends among the rustics in the Granite State, observing their ways.

As might be expected, visiting doctors who hear about bee-sting therapy warn its practitioners that they are risking a fatal reaction to the venom—which is indeed the case—and they usually dismiss the claims for its efficacy out of hand. But the claims persist. Following a hunch, several years ago Dr. Harold Clark in our laboratory sent away for some bee venom and our microbiologist, Jack Bailey, tested it against various strains of mycoplasma. It proved to be a very potent suppressor of their growth.

I am happy to report that the bee venom story isn't likely to end there. Some researchers in Great Britain have been studying its effects on arthritis and attempting to dissect it chemically, aiming toward the possibility that they will be able to separate the curative component from the part that creates the sting. It would be my own guess that the cure and the sting are one and the same thing, but I am delighted to see more research that is directed toward the mechanism by which arthritis occurs.

In the main, the history of arthritis research over the past four decades has been one of frustration, suffering, or serial disappointment as one miracle cure after another failed to live up to its early promise. The reason for those failures always comes down to one basic flaw: no major disease has ever been cured before science has first developed an understanding of how it works.

COMPLETING THE PUZZLE

At long last, the main parts of the puzzle are falling into place, and our understanding of the fundamental mechanism of rheumatoid arthritis is now nearly complete. There are still many aspects that need to be explored, but this new framework allows us to approach them in a different light, no longer dismissing the disease as hopeless and without a known cause.

This is the framework within which arthritis occurs. The process taking place within that framework is often far more complicated than I have shown, and some of its parts are still only dimly seen. There may well be other bacteria that contribute to the process of arthritis once it starts. Many people with tonsillitis or bad teeth or kidney infections may experience flares in their arthritis from these additional sources of antigen, just as people with noses that are sensitized to ragweed will find that they have also become sensitive to such other stimuli as house dust and feathers. But as surely as the primary cause of hay fever is ragweed, the starting point for arthritis is mycoplasmas.

Once a person's joints have become sensitized to mycoplasmas, which move in and settle there, other antigens can move into the same neighborhood and compound the problem. If there is a strong history of streptococcal infection (rheumatic fever, scarlet fever, frequent strep throats with ear and sinus complications) or a strongly positive ASO (streptococcal antibody level), additional treatment with appropriate antistreptococcal medication as a therapeutic probe is often indicated. Regardless of these other factors, however, the basis for the initial sensitivity is still mycoplasma, and if the mycoplasma can be removed, the sensitivity level of the rest of the body can be lowered as well and the other factors become more manageable. This framework provides the conceptual core for at last proving the cause of rheumatoid arthritis and finding its cure.

CHAPTER 19

How Do People Get Rheumatoid Arthritis?

Rheumatoid arthritis is an acquired disease, but the way people get it—and whether they get it—is determined by factors that are as complex as arthritis itself.

The principal complication is in the fact that rheumatoid arthritis involves a bacterial allergy. One of the characteristics of bacterial allergies is that the allergic process is so powerful, the body isolates the germ and keeps it from being transmitted to others.

A good model for that phenomenon is undulant fever, or brucellosis, a disease acquired from cattle or swine. Undulant fever is highly contagious among such livestock, and if one animal catches it, the disease spreads through the herd like wildfire. Man can contract undulant fever by drinking milk from an infected animal, but it has never been known in the history of medicine that the disease has been transmitted from one human to another. I believe the reason is that man, unlike cattle and swine, is so reactive to the antigens made by brucellae that the reactive state walls it off and keeps it highly localized, not allowing it to become a contagious entity. The same thing happens with mycoplasmas.

TWO KINDS OF IMMUNITY

There are two main types of immunity: bloodstream immunity, in which certain factors in the blood protect us against particular diseases, and cellular immunity, in which the same protection is provided by the tissues of the body. The lack of cellular immunity is the reason children contract measles, whooping cough, chicken pox, mumps, and other so-called childhood disorders.

We know that mycoplasmas can be recovered from the genital tracts of women as a matter of routine. We look upon these organisms as parasites at that stage, but their presence at the end of the birth canal creates the possibility of a scenario in which the child can become infected and the relatively passive parasitic mycoplasma can eventually be transformed into an active agent of disease. If it happens that the mycoplasma enters the infant's body, the parasite could escape into the bloodstream and be carried to the joints, where it would attach to the synovial cells. It could remain in the parasitic stage indefinitely, ticking away, awaiting its time to turn into something far more serious.

RAISING SENSITIVITY

As the years go by, it is possible that these and other factors raise the body's level of sensitivity until it finally reaches a point where, on a localized basis, the stage is set for an allergic reaction. The allergy would be the result of the body responding to the persistent presence of these organisms by raising a defense to surround them. How the reaction is triggered is the subject of speculation: it might be an accidental bump or contusion, or severe mental stress—or in some cases it might be the trauma of childbirth. I have treated a great many patients who never suspected they had any kind of arthritis until they had gone through some such seemingly unrelated shock or stress. Almost invariably they have associated their disease with the event that acted as the trigger.

LIKE A VIRUS

If this linkage is correct, as I suspect it is, then the mycoplasma acts in the same way as a slow virus. Once the liberating event has set it off, it begins to create a reaction that walls it off even further to defend itself against attack by the body's immune system. That would explain why as arthritis becomes more entrenched it also becomes more severe.

This scenario also supports the thesis that all the rheumatoid forms of arthritis derive from essentially the same causes, as I believe they do, and that the many variations in the disease are simply a result of differing levels of allergy and reactivity in the hosts. Similarly, people who suffer from asthmatic allergies may react to dust in one case and feathers and pollens in another, but the allergy itself, regardless of the source, is the cause of their distress.

SOME DISTINCTIONS

The analogy with asthmatic allergies only holds up to a point, however; rheumatoid arthritis involves a living source of antigen which cannot be isolated from the patient in the way of ragweed or feathers. Bacterial antigens appear to have a physiological effect on things inside the body such as joints, muscles, nerves, the intestinal tract, and internal organs. The internal allergy is generally referred to as hypersensitivity to distinguish it from external allergies. Ordinary allergies affect the skin, the lungs, the eyes, and generally the outside of the body. Both can affect an intermediate ground, the gastrointestinal tract. External allergies come and go with changes in the environment, such as the seasons, or simply with cleaning the house or filtering the air. But internal hypersensitivities are built in and they persist, and the antigen from a bacterial source keeps coming, constantly or intermittently, and serves as a booster.

The reason housecleaning doesn't work with internal allergies is that they are so inaccessible, and as these hypersensitivity conditions get worse they get even harder to reach because the walls around them rise progressively higher. When viewed under the microscope, the areas of inflammation in the affected tissues are seen to be spotty, as though the body had erected a series of tiny fortresses around the causative factor.

At the very center of those fortresses are the mycoplasmas. Although their presence can be verified by other means such as protein fractionation, they usually can't be seen with certainty even by an electron microscope; the particles are so tiny that they are indistinguishable from the parts of the cell to which they attach. Even when a tissue is deliberately inoculated with mycoplasmas and the physician examines electron-microscopic sections of the infected cells, it is difficult to determine which of the particles are derived from mycoplasmas and which represent normal cellular constituents. Little wonder that the mycoplasmas' relationship to rheumatoid arthritis has eluded understanding for so long.

This near-invisibility is one more respect in which mycoplasmas are different from any other kind of disease agent. Even viruses, which are equally small, have what are called nuclear inclusions; the inclusion body in the nucleus of the cell for certain viruses is very distinctive, lining up in a crystalloid pattern of specks, and this "fingerprint" of one virus will be recognizably different from the pattern of another. Mycoplasmas don't line up in the nucleus.

LUPUS AND OTHER RHEUMATIC DISEASES

It is my belief that all of the rheumatic disorders, from the mildest arthritis to the most fatal form of lupus, involve mycoplasmas as a causative agent. There are two possible reasons for the same cause to produce such widely differing results: there are variations in how strongly the different tissues react against the organism, and there are some forms of mycoplasma that are more virulent than others.

There are other reasons for the immense number of variables in the arthritis family tree. Once the focus of sensitivity is established by the unique ability of the mycoplasma to attach to joints, other bacterial antigens can enter the picture and compound the problem. This is particularly true of the streptococcal antigen, which has a special affinity for sensitizing joints, as in rheumatic fever. Infected teeth, tonsils, sinuses, gallbladders, kidneys, and diverticula can contribute and often must be treated separately.

PNEUMONIA AS TRIGGER

The most vicious strain of mycoplasma that has been isolated to date and one whose antibody is very commonly present in the blood of rheumatoid arthritics is *Mycoplasma pneumoniae*, which causes viral pneumonia. I don't have any statistics on its incidence, but a lot of my patients over the years—far above the norm for the population as a whole—have suffered from walking pneumonia, an event which may well have supplied the trigger for a sudden upsurge in their arthritis.

THE L-FORMS

Another dimension of the question about the causes of arthritis that deserves far more laboratory research is all the other L-forms of bacteria. The L-forms so closely resemble mycoplasmas in the laboratory that at one time all mycoplasmas were referred to as L-form bacteria. If a researcher grows streptococci on a laboratory medium, adds penicillin to the medium, and kills the strep or other bacteria, he may see tiny, microscopic colonies of what look like clusters of fried eggs emerging from the remains of the germ, in exactly the same manner as mycoplasmas produce such colonies.

Microbiologists claim these particular fried eggs are not identical to mycoplasmas, and indeed there are some chemical differences. But they are the same in form and structure, and are specifically suppressed by tetracycline derivatives, as are mycoplasmas. They behave the same way, growing on the surface of media. Protein fractionation, electrophoresis, and other study techniques are just now starting to provide valuable clues to their exact nature and relationship to the arthritic process.

The payoff on such research could be enormous. In rheumatic fever, for example, streptococcus splits off L-forms which very likely get into connective tissue in joints, the heart muscle, and even heart valves. One cannot grow the strep from the joints or heart muscle or valves, but it is possible the L-form is in these places, setting up a local sensitivity without the strep itself being present. If so, that would explain the chronic, destructive changes that go along with rheumatic fever. It is curious that the damage to the joints is not permanent, but clears up when the disease comes to an end. But the damage to the kidney or heart that has been caused by this unknown factor—a strep antigen or whatever—does not clear up, and it can shorten life.

I wouldn't be at all surprised if research were to prove that when the L-form becomes fixed as a new entity, it becomes a mycoplasma. Phylogenetically, this could mean that back at the beginning of life, millions of years ago, there were only bacteria, and some of them evolved into the L-forms which later became mycoplasma, and some of them went in another direction to become parasites, amoebas, and other such organisms, adapting to changes in the environment.

ALL CONNECTIVE TISSUE DISEASES CAN BE TREATED EQUALLY

All diseases of the connective tissue are related to the same process that controls the rheumatoid forms of arthritis, and all respond, in greater or lesser degrees, to the same antibiotic approach to treatment. Lupus, which is a disease whose mortality figures are extremely unreliable because of a lack of continuity in observation, may kill as many as 75 percent of those who contract it. I have had consistently positive results in treating even very advanced cases with tetracycline, including several patients who have now reached what appears to be permanent remission.

One connective-tissue disease that proves the case for tetracycline even more incontrovertibly is scleroderma. It is a chronic hardening and shrinking of the connective tissues in which the skin turns to leather and, because the blood vessels are involved as well, the extremities become numb and cold. It affects the ectodermal portion of the esophagus so that eventually the patient loses the peristaltic motion that permits swallowing, and it can even invade the lungs and intestinal tract. It is a slow, progressive, inevitable death.

During the past few years, I have been sent a number of scleroderma patients from Athens, Alabama. They have all tested high for mycoplasma antibody levels—just as patients with lupus or rheumatoid arthritis or mixed osteo-rheumatoid arthritis or dermatomyositis do—and I have treated every one of them with tetracycline, just as I treat everyone who is suffering from these or any other disease of the connective tissues. And the scleroderma patients have all improved, some dramatically.

In the case of scleroderma, any improvement at all is dramatic, but these improvements are truly remarkable. The patients have increased their ability to swallow. The skin on their face and hands has started to loosen up and become supple again. Those who have been caught early don't have any further progression of the disease, and those who started late have begun to reverse their condition. The most striking result has been the reversal of widespread sclerodermatous pulmonary lesions.

A lot of doctors like to explain away any progress in rheumatoid arthritis or lupus by calling it natural remission. But they can't explain what happens with scleroderma as a natural remission because with that disease there isn't any such thing: under any other form of treatment the disease only goes one way, downward, and it doesn't stop until the patient is dead.

PINNING DOWN THE MYCOPLASMA

All these different types of connective-tissue disorders involve a circulating antibody against mycoplasma, but that is not to say that every patient proves positive for those antibodies every time he or she is tested. In those cases where the results are negative, as a rule all that is required to get a positive result is to follow the patient for a period until the antibody pops up again. The process of antibody circulation in rheumatoid arthritis or other such diseases is very similar to that in undulant fever, which is often very difficult to diagnose because of the wavelike periodicity of the antibody. The cyclical appearance and disappearance of a disease antibody is a widely recognized phenomenon of immunology. The Herxheimer effect, which is a toxic surge that follows the onset of treatment for mycoplasmic disorders, brings out the antibody in patients who have tested negative prior to treatment; as the treatment progresses, the antibody eventually tests negative again.

Eventually there will be a test for the antigen of mycoplasmas as well as for the antibody; diagnosticians will be able to look for the disease factor that creates the condition, rather than seeking an indication of the body's response. This is an area of research in which the Arthritis Institute is vigorously active. We have also noted a greater concentration of both antigen and antibody in joint fluid compared to the blood serum from the same patient.

In order to identify the antigen, it is first necessary to break down tissue, joint fluid, or blood into its serial protein fractions. Blood has any number of different proteins in it, one of which turns out to derive from mycoplasma. We have been measuring the direct signs of mycoplasma in the blood—either its toxins, particles of the germ, or the entire disease organism—to see whether it goes away when the patient is treated intravenously with tetracycline. And we have shown that it does.

We have also been collecting and analyzing data to look for a correlation between the dropoff of the antigen and the status of the symptoms as the patient is treated. Preliminary data are not sufficient to prove anything significant, but there is enough positive evidence to encourage further effort. One of the benefits of such a correlation, if it is proven, will be to provide an alternative to double-blind testing.

Not all of the information that has developed from fifty years of research and practice with connective-tissue disorders is of a kind that lends itself to statistical summary. In fact, I often feel that the source that has weighed most heavily over the long term, in helping me to understand what is involved in these diseases and in recognizing their patterns, is the kind of data that scientists characterize as anecdotal. In time, as it repeats itself over and over again, anecdotal data becomes progressively more substantive and meaningful. Perhaps more than any other aspect of learning, it has provided the deepest insights into the process by which arthritis happens to people.

That is the principal reason for the approach we have taken in the writing of this book.

CHAPTER 20

Scleroderma: Two Stories

DOYLE BANTA
Preacher/Educator/Businessman
Athens, Alabama

One morning about seven years ago, I noticed something strange on the inside of my left leg, just below the big muscle. It was about the size of a dime and it looked like a scar. I couldn't remember ever having injured my leg there, and I studied it, trying to figure out what it was.

Some time later I was in Birmingham to see my doctor about a thyroid problem, and I thought to show it to him. He couldn't figure it out either, but he said he wasn't a dermatologist; he suggested I put a little Vaseline on it and watch it.

A few months later it was about the size of a quarter and still growing, and it had started to change color, to get darker. I went over to a dermatologist in Decatur, and he diagnosed me as soon as he saw it. I can say that I'm one of the few cases that ever got a diagnosis so soon; I've met a lot of people since then who have scleroderma, lupus, multiple sclerosis, rheumatoid arthritis, and other things like that, and every one of them got diagnosed with something else before their doctors finally got it right.

The doctor told me a couple of interesting things about scleroderma: he said it's a rare disease, that it's even rarer for someone my age to get it, and rarer yet because I am a man. Most victims are twenty to forty years old, and 80 percent of them are women. He said to me, "I'll bet you thought you had cancer."

I said, "Well, I've seen enough cancer patients in my life, and I did think that's what it was."

"No, it's scleroderma," he said. "I'm not going to biopsy it because the wound will never heal up. But that's what it is."

I asked him what we should do about it, and he told me we couldn't do anything. He said he didn't know of anyone who had ever gotten over it, and he didn't know any place I could go to see a doctor who could give me any help. "But I will tell you this," he said. "Before it's over, you're going to wish it had been cancer instead."

I asked him why he said that. I told him the little amount I had on my leg didn't hurt at all, and I had heard that cancer was really painful.

"This will hurt you just as much as cancer. But the thing about cancer is that in a relatively short time it will wipe you out. Scleroderma won't; if a person is in good enough shape to begin with, it can last for as long as ten years."

"You think I'm going to live ten years with this disease before it kills me?" I asked.

"Not at your age," he answered. "I think you're probably going to live another three to five. And I wish you luck. If you find anybody that can do anything to help you, I'd sure like you to let me know."

We didn't make any plan that I would go back to him, because there didn't seem to be any point in it.

I've been preaching for forty-eight years, I've been on the board of Florida College in Tampa for twenty-four years, I've taught here in Athens, I know a lot of people through my insurance business, and I've traveled all over the country—so I get to meet a lot of people. I started hearing about folks who knew other people who had the same disease I had, and I talked with a lot of them, trying to find out what they were doing about it. We compared notes on how they first heard about it, and what their symptoms were. We kept in touch, and as the disease got further along for each of us, we'd tell each other our symptoms.

Over the next three and a half years, my scleroderma got really bad. By the middle of 1984 I didn't have any feeling in either leg from the middle of my thighs down to the ends of my toes. The skin on both legs was as dark as shoe leather, and just as hard, from about six inches above my knees all the way down. The pain was getting worse and worse; at night, it got so severe I would jump out of bed and walk for a long time to try to get some activity in the legs and both feet. I came on the idea that maybe heat would help, and so I started sleeping with two or three pairs of socks and a heating pad, and that provided some relief, but things were still very bad. With scleroderma, the blood vessels get squeezed from the thickening of the skin and the circulation gets cut off. I was afraid they were going to have to amputate my legs.

Another thing happened to me at about the same time: I began to get rheumatoid arthritis. After a while it got so painful, especially in the joints of my hands, that it sometimes hurt more than the scleroderma did. My doctor started me on steroids.

I prayed a lot. I decided I'd like to live longer, since I had a wife and two children and a daughter-in-law and six little grandkids. One Saturday I went to Huntsville, which I seldom do, to visit a friend who was planning on doing some building there. And while I was standing in his store, in walked a boy that I went to college with in Abilene, Texas, in 1941, someone I hardly ever see. We started talking, and he asked if I knew that a good friend of ours from years ago was suffering from cancer. "Nope, I hadn't heard that, and I'm mighty sorry," I said.

We talked about our friend for a while, and then I said, "Well, I've got something that's supposed to be even worse, and that's scleroderma."

"Man," he said, "I have good news for you."

"What's that?" I asked.

"There's a lady here in town, a good friend of ours, who has the same thing. She went to see a doctor somewhere in the northeast, and now she's in remission."

The lady's name was Cathryn Loftis. He gave me her telephone number and I called her. She listened to my story and told me just what to do. I then called my doctor, my doctor called Dr. Brown, and Dr. Brown said he was booked up for a whole year. But my doctor said I was a good friend of his and I was awful sick, and Dr. Brown changed things around to make room for me; three weeks later I was sitting in his office at the National Hospital in Arlington, Virginia. It was May of 1984.

There have been lots of changes in my scleroderma since Dr. Brown began his treatment. The dark leather has retreated halfway down my legs to several inches below my knees and keeps on getting smaller. There is still a dark area on one leg about the size of my hand, but otherwise the dark spots have gotten lighter and in some areas have gone away. The real difference is that I'm still alive, and both my doctor in Alabama and I agree that I wouldn't be if I hadn't heard about Dr. Brown. I live a hectic schedule in connection with my preaching, my insurance business, and the school, and I'm able to keep up with all of it. I still have a way to go, but I believe I'm headed for remission.

I stayed in the hospital in Virginia for twelve days that first visit, and Dr. Brown treated my scleroderma intravenously. He had me come back again in the late fall for another twelve days, and for two twelve-day visits the following year. In 1986 I had an unrelated problem with a kidney blockage that kept me in Alabama that May, but it cleared up and I went back to Dr. Brown for another stay that December.

Between visits to the hospital, I continue the treatment at home. I have done tremendously well, and everybody who knows me is just amazed at how I've recovered.

Fortunately, I have a lot of friends, and one of the great joys

I have gotten out of this is that I've sent forty people to Dr. Brown in the past three years, not just the people I met who have scleroderma, but also people with lupus and with rheumatoid arthritis, and every one of them has come back home and done what he said and is getting better. I stay in touch with them by telephone, and I know they all are just as amazed as I was at how Dr. Brown is able to get them better when everyone else had pretty much given up on them.

It also still amazes me that everyone I talk with who has scleroderma tells me the same thing about the way their previous doctors treated them: they just diagnosed the disease, got them started on steroids, and sent them home to die. Everyone I have ever sent to Dr. Brown is still alive. Not one of the lupus or scleroderma patients has died, and it doesn't look like anyone is going to, at least not from those diseases.

I'll be sixty-eight years old in January. Today I look ten years younger than I did three years ago. My skin looks healthy. Three years ago I was just dragging around, and today I'm on the go more than ever. In addition to the scleroderma getting so much better, there isn't a single trace of rheumatoid arthritis left in my hands or anywhere else, and my joints look as good as they ever have in my life. Dr. Brown told me that scleroderma and rheumatoid arthritis are both caused by a germ called a mycoplasma, and the same treatment with tetracycline helps get rid of them both. He sure was right. It's unbelievable to me how many people I've met who were at the brink of death, and he's brought them back to a good life.

CATHRYN LOFTIS
Housewife, Huntsville, Alabama

In 1976, I developed hepatitis and my recovery was very slow. My doctor followed me closely, and he said he thought the reason the hepatitis was giving me so much trouble was that there was something else there as well, something that he hadn't identified. He ordered a liver biopsy, and the lab kept it for two weeks; they couldn't figure out what it was either.

The biggest symptom was my extreme fatigue. Most of the time I felt as though I had just run a marathon; if I got up at seven, by ten o'clock I'd have to go back to bed. It was a tremendous change from the way I used to be: I had played tennis a lot and was extremely active, and now I felt as though my head was in a vise and I walked around in a stupor. The doctor kept bringing me back for more tests and finally, after about a year and a half, he called me in one day and told me he thought I had a disease of the connective tissue.

I knew that wasn't good. A close friend of mine had a connective-tissue disease, one that affected all her muscles. The doctors had told her she had about seven years, and that was just about how long she lived.

One of the things the doctor noticed at that visit was that the skin on the ends of my fingers had gotten slick and unhealthy-looking. He asked me if I had noticed any changes in them over the past few months, and I had to admit I hadn't—I had been so distracted by my fatigue, I hadn't paid much attention to anything else. But my husband said that he saw the change, that the skin around the base of my fingernails seemed to be bowing out and that it had lost its natural color.

Our doctor sent me to a rheumatologist in Birmingham who examined me and said he thought I had an early case of scleroderma. By then the skin on my wrists was starting to thicken and I was seeing similar changes on either side of my face. That doctor sent me back to a dermatologist in Huntsville for a biopsy of one of the affected areas on my wrist. He told me to bring a picture of myself taken a year or more earlier, so there would be some basis for comparison in keeping track of the changes.

The dermatologist didn't want to do a biopsy when he first saw me, because he said he didn't think I had scleroderma. But after he looked more carefully at my face and hands he agreed there was some thickening so he went ahead. When he got back the lab report he told me he was sorry, that the test had been positive, and he sent me back to the rheumatologist.

When I heard that, I knew it was serious, and so I was prepared for the worst. But I got a very different story at my next visit to the rheumatologist. He told me he was going to start me on Naprosyn (a nonsteroidal anti-inflammatory), and that he was sure I was going to handle the disease beautifully. He said there was no sign that the scleroderma had gotten inside my body yet, and the treatment was starting early enough that it probably never would touch any of my internal organs.

My local doctor had asked me to call him when I got back, and when he heard what the rheumatologist had told me he said, "But that just isn't so! It *will* affect your major organs and it will get progressively worse." I trusted and respected him, and knew he was telling me the truth.

Just a short time later, my husband, Lewis, was reading the paper and he saw a story about a Dr. Thomas McPherson Brown who had been invited to lecture at the University of Alabama in Huntsville. The story said that Dr. Brown had had remarkable success in treating rheumatoid arthritis, and Lewis wondered if he might have some ideas about scleroderma, which was in the same family. The next day I called our family doctor, and his response surprised me. "Of course he would! Of course you should talk to him! I read all about Dr. Brown's lecture, and I don't know why I didn't put two and two together. There's no question he's on to something with arthritis, and he's just the person you should be talking to about scleroderma." He was very distressed with himself for not thinking of it first and calling us.

He offered to telephone the Arthritis Institute in Washington for us, and he called back a short time later to say that Dr. Brown did indeed treat scleroderma, that he had had a lot of success with it, and that my doctor had already told his nurse to send my records to the National Hospital. We made an appointment for me to be in Washington three months later.

Meanwhile, we began to hear some extraordinary things

about Dr. Brown from other people around Huntsville. Lewis came home one evening and told me that a secretary at the Arsenal who had had rheumatoid arthritis so badly she couldn't type anymore had been treated by Dr. Brown, and her disease had nearly disappeared. I later heard that the wife of one of our county commissioners had been so sick with rheumatoid arthritis that she was in bed and her husband even had to feed her. She had been taken to see Dr. Brown, and some months later a friend had called her. The phone rang a long time, and just as the friend was about to hang up the woman answered. She sounded wonderful, and when the friend apologized for bothering her, she said it was no bother at all—she had just walked into the house from a trip to do her Christmas shopping. In every case, we were told that the improvement didn't take place overnight, that it took a lot of patience, but that Dr. Brown got nearly incredible results.

By the time I kept my appointment in Washington, in June of 1978, the evidence of the scleroderma on both my face and hands had become much more pronounced. The affected areas were alternately sickly white or flushed an unhealthy pink; I could see what the doctor called "the butterfly" of the disease on my face. My cheekbones looked gaunt and the skin over them was stretched unnaturally tight. I couldn't tolerate temperature variations in either direction by more than a few degrees. The first two fingers of my right hand had turned virtually to stone; I could have stuck a knife into either of them and I wouldn't have felt a thing. My energy level was so low that all I could do in a day was get out of bed in the morning and put on my clothes, and housework was out of the question. When we finally met Dr. Brown that night after I had checked into the hospital, Lewis asked him, "What does my wife have to look forward to?"

Dr. Brown smiled reassuringly and said, "Everything."

He told us we had to be patient, that the treatment didn't work overnight—that it could even take years—but that we could expect me eventually to be able to lead a perfectly normal life.

Three days after I started the antibiotic therapy I was taking a shower at the hospital and the rings on my left hand suddenly slipped off the finger. I told Dr. Brown about it right away; I couldn't believe the tetracycline had already had such a powerful effect on the swelling of the scleroderma. He was pleased, but he told me the swelling would return and that I shouldn't be disappointed when that happened. He warned me that it would take a total of three years before I saw any really significant difference, and for the first six months of his treatment I was going to feel worse and I would test worse.

I'm not sure how much worse I really felt in the next six months, but there's no doubt he was right that I didn't get any better during that time. I was still terribly fatigued, and I had almost no energy for anything except getting up and going back to bed. When the six months were up I went back to Washington for more treatments and another set of tests, and sure enough the scores were worse than when I had entered the hospital for my first stay the previous June. But on the visit after that, also as Dr. Brown had predicted, the results began to improve. And it kept on like that. Two years and seven months after he had first treated me, I noticed a distinct change in the way I felt. I had more energy, I could stay up longer, I could do more things and I felt better. After that it was more good days and fewer bad days in a steady pattern of progress. The swelling stopped being a problem.

During my semiannual visit in December of the fourth year, Dr. Brown came into my room at the hospital and told me he had a Christmas present for me. He held up the test results he had just gotten back from the laboratory, and for the first time since I had been diagnosed with scleroderma, they were negative. The disease I had been told would kill me—that kills everyone who catches it—was in remission. More than that, it had reversed.

I am very grateful for what Dr. Brown has done, and I am also grateful to the doctor who brought us together—that he cared enough about me to be open-minded and willing to believe that someone else might have the answer when he and others did not. I have talked with a lot of people with scleroderma and arthritis and other connective-tissue diseases since then, and I know that not every doctor in America is that generous.

In the several years since that happy Christmas, my test results have remained absolutely normal, with no sign of the disease. It is now ten years since I was first diagnosed, and I have reached the limit of the longest possible life that someone with my original prognosis could expect to survive. The skin on my face and hands has returned to normal; the thickening and discoloration have disappeared and it has regained its original healthy elasticity. The circulation in my fingers is not all it might be, and my fingers sometimes get cold, but their full feeling has returned and there is no trace of the disease. Changes in climate or room temperature no longer bother me. I have as much energy as I had before I came down with the disease ten years ago. I walk three miles every day, feeling great every step of the way. I can do anything I want to do. I am fully recovered.

Just a little while ago a friend of mine discovered she had lupus. I told her to get right up to see Dr. Brown as fast as she could. She said she wanted to, but she was having a lot of trouble getting her dermatologist to send her records to the National Hospital; he said Dr. Brown was a quack. My friend told him that he had helped everyone she knew that had seen him, and that he even cured a woman who had scleroderma—referring to me, but not by name. The dermatologist laughed and said, "Nobody has ever cured scleroderma. If Dr. Brown helped your friend, then she didn't have scleroderma in the first place."

"Maybe not," my friend said, "but ten years ago you seemed to think she did. You were the one who diagnosed her."

CHAPTER 21

Doctors vs. Patients

We had a patient a few years ago who came to us from a university town in North Carolina. Before she got to us, she had been thoroughly poisoned with gold and cortisone, neither of which had worked; we treated her with tetracycline, and she did very well. She had some damaged fingers from her earlier intense rheumatoid arthritis, and when her disease had quieted down and she was feeling in good shape, she decided the time was right to get the fingers fixed. We talked it over and agreed she should go back to her hometown where there was a good hand surgeon connected with the university's medical school. A few weeks later she returned to Washington and told me this story.

When she had arrived at the office of the hand surgeon, he said he wanted her to see the rheumatologist at the university hospital. She explained that she already had a rheumatologist, but the surgeon insisted, saying that in cases involving rheumatoid arthritis, such referrals were "a matter of routine." So she made an appointment and went to see him.

The rheumatologist was the head of his department at the medical school and a very imposing figure. He exchanged a few pleasantries with my patient, then asked her what she was doing about her arthritis. She said, "Well, I see Dr. Brown in Arlington, Virginia. Do you know him?"

The doctor said, "I've heard of him. What is he giving you?"

"Tetracycline."

The rheumatologist recoiled. "That's terrible," he said. "He shouldn't be doing that."

She said, "It saved my life. My arthritis is under control for the first time in years, I've managed to get off the gold and cortisone before they killed me, and I'm doing fine."

The rheumatologist wasn't used to working with patients who really understood the nature of their medication or had the psychological energy to fight back, and he immediately retreated.

My patient, on the other hand, recognized a very familiar situation and was angry at this attempt to manipulate her. Moreover, she was the kind of lady who couldn't resist the opportunity to drive home an important point. "You know, doctor," she said, warming to her task, "I sat in your waiting room for nearly an hour before you could see me, and I had a chance to talk with a good number of your patients, most of whom tell me they have been coming to you for several years. I asked them the same question you just asked me: What are they doing about their disease? And they told me they are taking gold and cortisone. And do you know what impressed me most about those patients, Doctor? I don't believe I have ever seen such a gloomy, depressed, forlorn, and unhappy group of people in my entire life."

The doctor cleared his throat, probably in preparation to offer some kind of rejoinder, but my patient stood up cheerfully and extended her hand in farewell. "Goodness me, look at the time. I have a dinner date tonight with the chancellor of the university, and I have to run."

That was the coup de grace, and the doctor could barely rise to his feet. Somehow, he found the presence of mind to say, before she swept from the room, that he would like to see her one more time the following day. She very graciously agreed and they set the hour.

The next morning she kept her appointment, and unlike the day before the doctor saw her at precisely the specified time. His tone had changed remarkably. "I have been thinking about this all night," he said. "I believe you're doing very well with the treatment you're now getting, and I want to encourage you to keep it up."

The hand surgery went very well, and she is now free of arthritis and no longer takes medication of any kind.

IT'S NOT EASY BEING A RHEUMATOLOGIST

Doctors don't like patients who complain, and they don't like them sitting out there in the waiting room, advertisements for failure. In the field of arthritis, a subtle antagonism has developed between many doctors and their patients because of this, more than in any other field of medicine. It is not at all uncommon for patients to tell me that their previous doctor has said, "Your problem is that you can't take pain," or "It's a shame you can't take my medicine, which has been so helpful to others," or in some other way admonished them to stand up to the disease and learn to live with it. Of the 37 million stories of arthritis in America today, there are precious few in which the physician is willing to predict a happy ending. What they forecast instead, in many cases, is a gradual process of deterioration that will end in a wheelchair or a bed, with a great deal of pain.

If that situation makes the doctors angry, it makes the patients even madder. I asked one patient, from Huntsville, Alabama, why she had left her previous doctor. "Well, he had tried everything else and none of it worked," she said, "and so one day he told me he was going to try methotrexate. I'd heard that methotrexate was dangerous, and so I asked him the simple, obvious question: What had his experience been with risks from this drug? And he was so offended that he stood up, threw a syringe at me, and walked out. I walked out, too, and don't plan to go back."

It isn't uncommon for a doctor in this field to shed the patients that are difficult to deal with or who otherwise give him trouble, at the same time as he tries to collect well-to-do patients and stay as far as possible from anyone who looks like Medicare or Medicaid. The arthritics of the country aren't getting a fair shake. The rheumatology profession is one of weeding out: when a drug isn't working well or the patient is becoming more and more difficult to treat, the doctor would just as soon see him or her go someplace else.

THE SPIDERWEB

Rheumatology is a branch of medicine that works on the principle of the spiderweb. The specialist sits in the middle of the web, waiting for the general practitioners in his area to refer patients. It is a delicate art, because during this same process, the impression is created in the community that the general practitioner isn't good enough to treat arthritis.

Once the patient arrives in the rheumatologist's office, a course of treatment begins, usually with aspirin, then the nonsteroidal anti-inflammatory drugs and things of that sort. When they run out, then the patient is moved on to gold, Plaquenil, and penicillamine, and finally the immunosuppressive drugs such as Imuran and methotrexate. The whole procedure takes from two to five years, and then the point is reached where nothing works. When that finally happens, some rheumatologists simply roll over their list and send their patients back to the family practitioners who referred them in the first place. The standard phrase they use at this point is, "I'm sorry, but you can't take my medicines." It subtly places the responsibility back on the patient. And it is designed to create the impression that each patient who arrives at that condition is the only one it ever happened to, that he or she is hopelessly different. In fact, this may be the one respect in which every rheumatoid arthritic is the same: sooner or later, they all run out of medicine that works—if they live long enough—unless their physician puts them on a regimen of treatment that addresses the cause of their illness.

And this rollover process is going to continue until that happens.

One reason it may happen soon is Lyme disease.

Lyme disease looks a lot like rheumatoid arthritis. Unlike rheumatoid arthritis, however, there is a general agreement about its cause, and as a result, less than twenty years after it was first diagnosed Lyme disease now has a cure. And there is a feeling in the air that maybe rheumatoid arthritis has a knowable cause as well.

The road back has been defined, and it lies clearly before us.

CHAPTER 22

John Sinnott, D.O., Ida Grove, Iowa

I first came in contact with Dr. Brown's treatment several years ago through the family of a young arthritis patient here in Iowa named Don Knop. Don's folks were in the cattle business, and they heard about Dr. Brown from a woman they knew from somewhere down south who had been successfully treated by him. The family was weighing whether to send Don to the National Hospital in Washington, and they asked for my opinion.

I had to admit I knew nothing about Dr. Brown, so they gave me some tapes and articles about his approach. Everything I heard and read about the infectious nature of arthritis made good sense to me and was consistent with the things I had observed or suspected about the disease in the course of my own practice. So I did some checking in the Washington area, and learned that Dr. Brown was very highly regarded, and I recommended to the family that they send Don out to see him.

Don got better. A lot of people around here heard about it, and they asked me to send them to Washington for the same treatment. When they went, they got better, too. In a little while, it seemed that everybody in northwest Iowa and the whole Midwest was calling me up and asking me to refer them to the National Hospital. I couldn't send people I didn't know, so the Knop family asked why I didn't invite Dr. Brown out here to talk to area doctors and tell them how they could do the same thing themselves.

He came out in the summer of 1979, which was when I met him for the first time. He told me I should use his method in my own practice. When I asked him out, I had no intention of getting into that kind of treatment myself and I didn't know if I wanted to; I wasn't sure if I could or should. But he convinced me to try it. After I proved that it could work on the patients I already had who suffered from rheumatoid arthritis, I quickly found that I couldn't deny it to the other patients who started coming to me because they had heard about my results. My practice in arthritis suddenly mushroomed.

Dr. Brown's technique has been far more successful than anything I had done previously to help patients with rheumatoid arthritis and the results are better than any I have heard about elsewhere. I am satisfied that in the course of using his method I have not caused any of my patients harm, which is one of the first things that doctors who treat patients for arthritis have to think about.

I haven't done any research on my results, but I would estimate that up to about 85 percent of the patients I have treated this way have improved substantially. The remaining 15 percent represent patients whose disease was so far advanced, so aggressive, or so stubborn that I was not able to get the results I would have liked. I have always wished I lived closer to Dr. Brown so I could see how he would have handled these cases, but of course that's why I'm treating arthritics in the first place—because we live so far from the Arthritis Institute that the patients just can't get there.

As another guess, I would conservatively estimate that I have treated around two hundred patients with Dr. Brown's technique. The tradition of rheumatoid arthritis is that it's a discouraging disease and that patients don't get over it. I practice in a part of the country where people have to travel long distances, sometimes thirty miles, just to see their family doctor. There isn't any easy way to have follow-up under those circumstances, and patients don't drive that kind of distance without a good reason. I'm always amazed, even today, when I run into patients who I haven't seen in a few years and I ask them how they're doing and they say they're just fine, that the disease hasn't given them a bit of trouble in all the time since I last saw them. If I were using any other approach, I'd be pretty sure that the reason I hadn't seen them was that the treatment had failed, and not that it was such a success.

Quite a few people come to me because they have heard I'm getting good results with arthritis, and whenever someone like that walks in I make it a point to tell them I'm not an arthritis specialist, that I'm a general practitioner. The reason I do this is to let them know this isn't a dangerous technique that only a few doctors can handle, but that it's something any family practitioner can do. I tell them that if they have something requiring a specialist they should see one, but there are times when a specialist isn't necessary and this is one of them—it's so safe, even a country doctor like myself can do it.

I wish I could say that I haven't had any bad results using this approach, but that isn't the truth. My bad results—the *only* bad results—have been that Blue Cross/Blue Shield and Medicare refuse to give any recognition to this form of treatment. That's why I've lost contact with a lot of these patients; they can't afford to come back because the payment for follow-up comes right out of their pocket, and if there's nothing wrong they don't want to pay to have me to verify that they're well.

All the patients I've treated for rheumatoid arthritis have paid out of their own pockets, but there have been a lot more who turned away because they couldn't afford it, especially if it meant going into the hospital for intravenous therapy. The ones that don't have the money have been forced to find a doctor who would treat their disease with the standard arthritis medicines—treatments that cost much more, are highly dangerous, and will eventually fail—because that's the only way they can get anything under their insurance policies. And that really bothers me.

At first, Medicare wouldn't pay for the treatment because they said the approach was experimental. I've got all the paperwork showing the results with my own patients, and I've shown them all of Dr. Brown's results as well, including published research. So then they switched over to saying it's just investigational, because it's only done in a few widely scattered places around the country and hasn't been accepted nationwide as the standard treatment. It's Catch-22.

There's nothing worse than getting hopeful telephone calls from people on Medicare who are willing to drive several hundred miles to my office so I can give them some help with the pain and suffering of their rheumatoid arthritis—and having to tell them not to come because they can't afford the cost of the hospital. I won't start treatment unless I know I can get them on intravenous therapy if they need it, and most of the really bad cases do need it. It's a situation that just has got to change.

On the other side of the coin, a lot of the people who do start treatment with me are early enough in their disease that they can get good results fast. These are frequently people who have been diagnosed by other doctors and are smart enough to read up on the standard treatments before they begin; they discover that gold can be lethal and that other standard treatments can cause blindness or death, so they call me instead. Those are the people I treat and then might not see again for a couple of years until they drop by and tell me how well they are, that the arthritis is all gone. Those are the ones that make me feel good.

I suppose that if I had never met Dr. Brown, the number of arthritics I would treat in the normal course of my practice would only be about 5 percent of the number I see now. But even today the number of my arthritic patients would be a lot higher if I didn't have to turn so many away—people who are old and who Medicare won't pay for, people who are so sick they can't get here on their own, all looking for a little hope that I can't give them.

Eventually, this will change; in fact, I have seen some interesting changes already. In the time since I started using Dr. Brown's treatment, the attitude of my peers, including area rheumatologists and orthopedists, toward his infectious theory and the use of antibiotic therapy has shifted noticeably. The jokes and the snide comments have tapered off or come to an end. Other doctors read the same literature I do, and it's becoming pretty clear that the other avenues of treatment are coming to a dead end. As that happens, acceptance of the theory of an infectious source gets greater every day.

As good as it is, I'm sure that what I'm doing today is not the final answer. Dr. Brown has done almost all the work to get us to this point, and I'm certain he agrees with me that out of that groundwork there has to be an even better way to deal with this disease, one that will put it away for good for everyone. And I think he has brought us within reach of that happening.

CHAPTER 23

Rheumatoid Arthritis and Your Family Doctor

Just a few years ago, I was invited to Sweetwater, Tennessee, to talk about rheumatoid arthritis with staff doctors from the community hospital as well as other physicians from the area. My host had been a patient at the Arthritis Institute, had done well, was a member of the board of the hospital, and was concerned that there was no program of antibiotic therapy in that part of the country. There was a pretty good turnout for the meeting, partly because I told the doctors that I would be happy to look at any of their patients that they wanted me to see after the meeting.

I was particularly pleased that many of the doctors in that session were family practitioners. These days, family practitioners are very well trained in a qualification program that involves three years of hospital work, and they are capable of doing far more for patients than the general practitioners of a generation earlier. There are three reasons I feel that family practitioners are the best source for the treatment of patients suffering from rheumatoid arthritis: they are the physicians most likely to detect the disease early; they are inclined by their training toward safe remedies; and they are in the best position to provide continuity of care.

DR. CASEY

One of the family physicians who took me up on my offer was a Dr. Robert Casey, a young physician starting in family practice. After the general meeting we went to his clinic and he introduced me to a young farmer who had rheumatoid arthritis. I learned that the patient was about thirty, had a wife and four young children, and ran a successful farm in a nearby community. When I questioned him, the farmer told me he was ready to give up, and it was clear that he was terribly despondent.

He told me he had been to visit a rheumatologist in Knoxville, and that he had been on various remedies that had each, successively, failed to hold up and had made him sick. He said he was weak and tired, and that the strength had left his hands. As a farmer he needed his hands for just about everything, and he had reached the point at which he couldn't even hold on to the steering wheel of his tractor because of the weakness and pain. He said he planned to sell the farm.

In addition to wanting to help the patient for his own sake, I recognized right away that the case had all the elements to make a good demonstration for the local community of how well the basic treatment approach works. In rural areas, people tend to talk more with their neighbors than in cities, and I knew that word would get around that there was a safe, simple, inexpensive treatment for rheumatoid arthritis that really cured the disease.

Dr. Casey knew nothing more about the treatment than he had learned at our session earlier that same day, and because I worked miles away from Tennessee we all knew that I would not be available for future meetings with his patient. That was another positive aspect of this case as a model; it would be obvious to all the other physicians in the area that I wasn't stacking the deck by picking a doctor who knew everything I knew about rheumatoid arthritis and mycoplasmas. I told Dr. Casey and his patient about my plan, and they both agreed to give it a try.

I outlined a method of treatment, which included Dr. Casey calling me every couple of weeks to advise me on the patient's progress. I told the patient that he would have to hang in there for about six months, and that he would have very little encouragement during that period to indicate that good things were happening; he wouldn't feel much better, and he would still have the pain and weakness in his joints. It was a severe case. I asked, "Are you willing to fight a long battle if you know that there will be some signs of hope at the end of six months?"

He thought about it for a while, then said he would.

I also told him to find somebody in the neighborhood to give him some help with his work, that above all else he should keep the farm. "It's your livelihood, it's your future, and it's your family's future," I said. "You've got to hang on to it."

He agreed to that as well.

We started him on the program, which included some intravenous treatment to speed up the process. I no longer recall the details, but most likely it involved 250 milligrams of oral tetracycline three times a week, along with some low levels of anti-inflammatory drugs to relieve the pain, supplemented with an intravenous drip of tetracycline once every two weeks during his regular clinic visits.

As the weeks went on, Dr. Casey reported to me periodically that the patient seemed to be improving, after an initial worsening of symptoms. I asked about his spirits, which had previously been very depressed, and Casey said he thought they were picking up as well. There may have been some small adjustments to the treatment as it went along—if so, I no longer recall them—but at the end of six months Dr. Casey reported to me that the patient was almost completely well.

One of the reasons that the recovery was so dramatic is that men respond to treatment more quickly than women do. I have no idea why. Although there are exceptions on both sides, as a rule even the worst cases of rheumatoid arthritis in men show great progress in six months, and it takes women with the same degree of involvement about a third to half again as long to get to the same point. However, the difference between the sexes is not as important a factor as the length of time the patients have had the infection; the longer they have suffered from it and the more therapeutic failures they have had, the longer the time to get rid of it. There are so many other variables that I can seldom be certain just how long treatment will take, and I never promise the patient a final result by a given date. I tell them instead, "I know you are going to be all right eventually, but I don't know how long that is. Are you willing to go down this road?"

The time factor is an important consideration in starting a patient on antibiotic therapy, and it has to be handled properly at the beginning of treatment. Some doctors are concerned that they will lose their patients unless they can produce some results right away. This is the worst possible strategy: to risk the patient's well-being or even his life in exchange for short-term results. It has been my experience that when the timing is explained realistically, the patient is glad to make a commitment and stick with it to reach the sought-for remission.

As a result of his success with the young farmer, Dr. Casey decided to come to Arlington and spend a week with me at the Arthritis Institute. In the meantime, the farmer himself had been telling everyone who would listen how great the treatment was and how it had improved his life. Dr. Casey went back to Tennessee with a lot more specialized experience in treating the disease, and the Sweetwater Hospital set aside a section just for his use in working with rheumatoid arthritics.

By now Dr. Casey was getting a lot of referrals and repeating his success with arthritics from all over that part of Tennessee. He told me he had some misgivings about whether a family practitioner should be treating such a specialized practice, so with my encouragement he contacted leaders within the state Academy of Family Practice as well as educators in the discipline, including his former department head at the teaching hospital in Knoxville where he had completed his residency. He posed the question of whether it was an appropriate thing for him to be doing. Everyone he contacted told him they thought is was just fine, that the only criterion was whether the patients were achieving good results with little risk. I was impressed with that response; clearly, it put the needs of the patient first.

TETRACYCLINE THERAPY IS ABSOLUTELY SAFE

The reason I was able to work with Dr. Casey—and over the years with many other doctors who were a long distance away and whose patients I never met—was that we were dealing with a treatment that was absolutely safe. Tetracycline has been used for a long time in two chronic conditions without ill effect: bronchiectasis in old people and acne in the young. It would have been impossible to do this same thing with any of the kinds of therapy that are usually prescribed for rheumatoid arthritis, because they involve such substantial risk to the patient. At the outset, the process requires explanation and it needs guidance. Dr. Casey got to the point where he had a real instinct for the mechanism, and from there on he didn't need any further help.

Some patients are more sensitive than others to medication, and part of learning how to work with tetracycline is developing a reliable feel for how much is right in each case. This is made much easier by the fact that the dosage level which a patient accepts best is also the level that works best therapeutically; it isn't a matter of sensitive patients missing a part of the benefits because they need more tetracycline than they can handle.

Patients who react poorly to one form of tetracycline will frequently respond well to another. It is a drug that has been around long enough to be available in lots of forms. We have found, for example, that patients who do not respond well to tetracycline are often favorably responsive to oxytetracycline, a compound that is nearly identical chemically, or the other mycin drugs such as erythromycin, Vibramycin, or clindamycin. If there is a strong streptococcal history or a high level of antibodies against the streptococcus, ampicillin may have to be introduced. The main point is for the physician to gain a complete understanding of this mechanistic approach to guide his individualized strategy through the shifting terrain of rheumatoid arthritis. The doctor has to recognize that he is dealing with a very delicately balanced condition. It is a lot like walking through the woods in the dark; if you're on familiar ground and can recognize the landmarks as they pass underfoot, you get where you want to go—and if you miss, you run into the trees.

One of the problems with arthritis is that many of its victims can't tolerate any kind of oral medicine because their stomachs have become extremely reactive through long and escalating sensitization from many different medicines. Patients who may experience upset from taking tetracycline orally are likely to find that they have no such reaction when they start taking it intravenously. A third choice is intramuscular injection in the form of clindamycin; it is somewhat less effective than intravenous, but it's an alternative for patients whose blood vessels are hard to reach. (Someday, I expect we will see an antimycoplasma medication in a form that can be administered rectally, so it goes directly into the bloodstream without aggravating the oversensitized stomach.)

Family physicians are no strangers to monitoring and managing these kinds of variables as they treat the entire range of health problems they face daily. In most cases, they quickly master the subtleties of finding the most effective combination of form, dosage, and methodology for successful antibiotic therapy. They are careful not to use dangerous drugs. A busy practitioner simply does not have the time to monitor risky medications. Until now, the rheumatologist's role was essentially to guard against kidney, retinal, bone marrow, liver, and lung damage. The requirements of his vigil narrowed down the likelihood of reaching more than a handful of the 37 million arthritics in our country. With a safer method of treatment and a proper understanding of the disease mechanism, all patients can be reached, including the mixed osteo and rheumatoid arthritics, and at a quarter of the present cost.

CHAPTER 24

Hon. Thomas C. Reed

After serving as secretary of the Air Force during the Ford Administration, I returned to my construction and land development business in the spring of 1977—and in transit I took a long skiing vacation in Breckenridge, Colorado. During that vacation, I hurt my shoulder in a fall.

I didn't pay much attention to it at first; it was sore but not particularly painful, and I expected it would take care of itself as those things do. I was in my mid-forties, and when the soreness persisted, I assumed it just meant I had reached an age when that kind of thing takes a little longer. But it got steadily worse.

That summer I took my family out to our house in California. I like to swim, but every time I got into our pool the pain in my shoulder was more severe than the last, and I finally decided to give in to it and see about getting it fixed.

I went to our family doctor. I've always liked him; he's good at spotting problems, he isn't someone who makes a big deal out of a little one, and he has a good record for getting me back on my feet fast. He examined me thoroughly and said I probably had a touch of something like bursitis—but that what it really came down to was simply that I was getting older. If you have that kind of a fall in your mid-forties, you don't expect to bounce the way you did when you were twenty. He told me to let nature take care of it, and in the meantime to be careful not to do anything that might hurt the shoulder further. He also said I might eventually want a shot of cortisone, and he gave me the names of a couple of rheumatologists if the problem continued to get worse.

The problem did continue to get worse, but I was extremely busy and didn't take the time to do anything further about it for another several months. By that fall it had become very difficult for me to lift my arms over my head to put on a sweater, take a shower, or do anything else that required that kind of motion. It also slowed me down at work. I was trying to pick up my business again after working for the government, and I found myself hurting every time I reached up to get something out of a file. Business trips were a big part of my life, and they became an ordeal in which I knew I would have to endure several hours of aches, twinges, and stiffness.

In early November I spoke about it with my uncle Lawrence Reed, and he recommended that I see Dr. Brown over at the National Hospital.

Probably the thing that decided me was a trip we had scheduled with the kids. We had chartered a boat in the Caribbean for the Thanksgiving vacation, and as I looked forward to it I kept thinking how difficult it was going to be for me to swim and dive and do the other things we usually did on those trips with my shoulder in that condition. I gave Dr. Brown a call and went over to see him.

He had ordered some blood tests first, so by the time I got to meet him he already knew what was going on and was able to tell me exactly where I stood. He said I had tested positive for rheumatoid arthritis and that the trouble I was having with my shoulder wasn't going to get better if I continued to ignore it.

He told me what was involved in the disease—what causes it and how it can be successfully treated—and I have to admit that I learned more about mycoplasmas that day than I really wanted to know. My immediate purpose in going to him was to get fixed up so I could go sailing. I had no idea before then what a truly terrible disease rheumatoid arthritis can be.

Dr. Brown also told me about depression—that it was as much a part of rheumatoid arthritis as the pains and stiffness, and that it would go away with the rest of the symptoms as a result of his treatment. That wasn't something I had discussed with anyone else, but I was certainly aware that my spirits had been low as a result of the problem in my shoulder.

He started me off on aspirin to reduce the pain, along with intravenous treatments with an antibiotic, a form of tetracycline. He also told me that I wasn't going to be immediately better as a result of the treatment, and certainly not in time to get rid of the pain before I went sailing. He said it would be a gradual process, but that one day I would notice that it was starting to improve.

I remember Dr. Brown telling me that, because that's pretty much how it turned out. There was a total of about five intravenous treatments, spaced progressively further apart for a period of perhaps five months, along with daily doses of Clinoril (a nonsteroidal anti-inflammatory) and a couple of tetracycline tablets twice a week. I did go sailing with the family as planned, but as far as the arthritis was concerned it was an ordeal.

One day after about five months I was in the shower and when I reached up to get something, I realized the pain was completely gone. I said to myself, "It's all over. Amazing." I used up the rest of the pills Dr. Brown had given me but didn't bother to refill the prescription.

Things went along fine for a couple of years. In 1983, I began to get some of the familiar aches, stiffness, and twinges.

It wasn't as serious as the first incidence of arthritis, but once you've been hit between the eyes by a two-by-four, you look twice when you see someone down the street holding the same kind of board. So I headed right back to Dr. Brown. He did the usual blood tests and started me on the pills again. This time the arthritis went away in less than eight weeks.

Despite the fact that I can remember a particular event that made me aware my arthritis had left me the first time, I know that isn't the way the disease usually ends. It isn't like a bell going off to let you out of class or a tooth being pulled that cures the toothache. But there are moments—and they recur more frequently as you keep improving—when you realize you have regained your cheerful outlook on life, when you can pour a cup of coffee without getting a pain in your wrist and you can take a normal shower. Eventually those moments become continuous, and you realize it's over.

For the past three years I have taken no medication whatever and have remained totally free of any symptoms of rheumatoid arthritis. My energy level is as high as it has ever been, my spirits are up where they should be, I can travel without stiffness, swim without pain, and lead a normal life that is full and productive. Dr. Brown describes this as remission, because that's how doctors talk about a good result.

I call it a cure.

CHAPTER 25

How Tetracycline Works

When I first started working on rheumatoid arthritis at the Rockefeller Institute in the late 1930s, I decided to retrace a path that had been well worn by earlier investigators; I went to the joint fluid, looking for any signs of an infectious agent.

It was already established that regular bacteria don't operate in those parts of the body; such bacteria are hard to miss, and hundreds of earlier investigators had failed to isolate any infectious agent from the joint fluid of an arthritic. That didn't rule out regular bacteria as causative factors, but if streptococci were involved, for example, they apparently worked by setting up a command post elsewhere in the body—in a gland, probably—and telegraphing their effects, via toxins, to the afflicted areas. What I was looking for was some smaller organism, closer to the size of a virus, that lived and worked right in the joint.

SABIN'S MOUSE

It happened that Albert Sabin was working in a laboratory just down the hall at the time, studying a central nervous system disease called toxoplasmosis. One day he told me he had cultured the brain of a mouse and come up with a strain of mycoplasma. He said he nearly missed it; when he smeared the culture out and tried to stain it, he couldn't see anything, but something was clouding the media and he knew that some kind of organism was growing there. When he finally identified it as a mycoplasma, he put some of the cloudy culture fluid in a hypodermic and injected another mouse. As a result, the second mouse came down with a case of arthritis.

At the same time, I had succeeded in isolating a mycoplasma organism from the joint fluid of a human. For some reason, it was much more difficult to work with than was the mouse strain of mycoplasma. In later years, our work with gorillas and elephants would support those early observations that the mycoplasma strains associated with more complex immune systems in the higher animals are more difficult to isolate and study, although exactly why is still unknown.

The main area from which it was possible to recover mycoplasmas was the genital tract. When I got back to Johns Hopkins, I worked with specialists there and got cultures from the cervix in females and prostatic secretions in men, cultured them, and found mycoplasmas. Those strains had in common with the strains from Sabin's mouse cultures that they were susceptible to the same gold and quinine drugs that have an effect on arthritis. There was an obvious connection between mycoplasmas and arthritis in humans, just as Sabin had found there was in mice.

LOOKING FOR LOW-RISK ALTERNATIVES

Because the long-term risks were so much more substantial than any short-term benefits, I didn't want to use gold or Plaquenil to treat my arthritis patients. I started looking at all sorts of antibiotics for alternatives. Working with a brilliant, enthusiastic research fellow from Harvard named Jack Nunemaker whom the head of my department at Hopkins assigned to my project, I soon found there was one class of antibiotics that worked on mycoplasmas, and that was tetracycline, the so-called mycin group. The group included Aureomycin, Terramycin, Achromycin, lincomycin, erythromycin, Vibramycin, and clindamycin.

If mycoplasmas were difficult to isolate, in theory they would be even more difficult to eradicate, since they were either intercellular or under a great deal of inflammatory tissue. Because of that difficulty, I had no hesitancy about relentlessly pursuing the treatment with Aureomycin. If one were to think of rheumatoid arthritis as an ordinary infection, common sense would say to quit treatment if the patient didn't become well within a few days. But if the disease were viewed instead as a bacterial allergy, common sense would say to persist. That recognition of the true nature of the disease was an important turning point in understanding how it could eventually be subdued.

TETRACYCLINE IS NOT LIKE OTHER ANTIBIOTICS

The persistent use of tetracycline in pursuit of an infectious allergy ran against the common view of how antibiotics should be applied. Antibiotics were generally regarded at the time as a short-term response, used to treat pneumonia, strep throat, and other bacterial disorders, and were never used over an extended period because of the risk that the patients would develop immune strains of the germ for which they were being treated. This view was softened somewhat in more recent years by the discovery that some problems, particularly acne in children and bronchiectasis, a chronic affliction of older people marked by paroxysmic coughing, could only be cured by using antibiotics for a long time. But generally the expectation remains that antibiotics should produce results quickly, and if they don't, then the doctor should try something else.

TETRACYCLINE DOES NOT GIVE RISE TO IMMUNE STRAINS OF GERMS

The prolonged use of most antibiotics can indeed give eventual rise to an immune strain of germ. Immunity is developed in a germ's outer surface, which is the area affected by penicillin and other antibiotics. Tetracycline is different from all other antibiotics in that critical respect: it affects the core of the germ, not the outer surface, and therefore no immune strain of germs ever develops as a result of its use. Moreover, people who use tetracycline over a period of months or years tend to avoid colds, pneumonia, and other diseases.

Once the view of arthritis as an infectious allergy relieved us of the pressure for those immediate results, we were able to shift our attention to various manipulative techniques for increasing its effectiveness under varying conditions. Oral treatment worked just fine in relatively early cases, for example, where the degree of inflammatory reaction or obstruction by scar tissue had not had the opportunity to build up; longer-standing cases responded far better to intravenous treatment. These facts, too, supported the concept of the mechanism as we were coming to understand it.

GETTING WORSE, THEN GETTING BETTER

The Herxheimer phenomenon was further evidence that rheumatoid arthritis involved the release of an antigen or toxin rather than the more common disease process of a broad-scale bacterial invasion. I noticed in the beginning that when treatment was started with antibiotics, as many as 80 percent of the recipients got worse before they got better, indicating that the treatment was hitting a susceptible source.

It is interesting to note that the Herxheimer effect does not occur when one is treating a streptococcal infection with a penicillin derivative. The streptococcus is not located at the site of the irritation, is not protected by a barrier of inflamed or scarred tissue, and it is knocked out in the faster, more conventional manner of regular bacterial infections.

We know that tetracycline works on mycoplasmas specifically, and to a lesser extent on streptococci, but doesn't have a particular effect on other bacteria. Further, conventional bacteria would not be controllable by any antibiotic that was administered intravenously only once every two weeks or once a month. The reason for that broad period with tetracycline is to avoid a build-up of sensitivity to the drug so the body won't block its action against the mycoplasmas.

Because the process is a bacterial allergy, this approach works very well. By contrast, treatment of pneumonia with an antibiotic requires a round-the-clock assault on the pneumococcus germ in order to keep it suppressed until the body can take over and get rid of it; in that case, treatments spaced two weeks apart would simply allow the bacteria to build up again and come back stronger than ever. With a bacterial allergy, by contrast, the germ creates a little wall around itself, a tiny zone of toxin, which keeps the disease-fighting antibodies from reaching it; the therapeutic approach with tetracycline is simply to suppress the toxin, which is the germ's means of defense. The fact that tetracycline works in precisely that manner when used on rheumatoid arthritis is further proof of the infectious nature of the disease; if therapy is administered intermittently or unevenly, the results are intermittent or uneven in the same pattern. The same logic that linked mycoplasmas with arthritis in Sabin's mouse also proves the presence of mycoplasmas in humans when tetracycline is used as a therapeutic probe.

When tetracycline is used to suppress the toxin, the disease is eventually driven into remission. When it is not, the toxin enables the germ to stay in its host for twenty, forty, or sixty years—unless, of course, the host succumbs in the interim to some other form of treatment.

CHAPTER 26

A Physician's Guide to the Use of Tetracycline in Rheumatoid Arthritis

When a doctor starts any course of treatment that affects the antigen of this disease, he has to keep in mind that the tissues of the arthritic are very reactive and do not like medicines very much—but neither do they require much. The doctor also has to keep in mind a conceptual view of the disease process during treatment. An early case will accept medicine much better than a late one. A case in which the rheumatoid factor is negative is very much easier to treat than one in which it is positive. In either case, treatment cannot begin by throwing the book at a patient. Generally it starts by giving medication twice a week.

The allergic state in itself is anti-germ. This is an extremely important point. Sir William Osler, the great physician-in-chief at the Johns Hopkins Medical School at the turn of the century, observed that asthmatics were immune to getting pneumonia. He based that conclusion on the terrible epidemic in Philadelphia in which around a third of the population died of lobar pneumonia; the asthmatics came through that epidemic scot-free, although one might reasonably have expected that they would be among the first to go. When I was at Johns Hopkins some years later, I heard of Osler's observation and it amazed me. I tried to understand why that could be the case.

When the opportunity presented itself, I got some sputum from an asthmatic and looked at it for bacteria. Under the microscope it appeared to be sterile. I got some cultures, and nothing grew. Osler had been right; there is something in the asthmatic's system that is anti-germ.

I tried to imagine what it could be. We knew that asthmatics produce histamine, which causes the bronchial tree to go into spasms. The histamine figures in an allergic reaction which is very delicately poised; pollen or some other irritant comes along and the muscles in the bronchial tubes squeeze down and contract. But that didn't explain the sterility. I filed the phenomenon away in my mind and went on to other things.

When I started in arthritis research at the Rockefeller Institute, the clinical side of the institute was a hospital for special diseases. I took care of a ward in the institute hospital that was filled with children with rheumatic fever. We knew that rheumatic fever was due to streptococcus; the first person to type out the streptococcus was Rebecca Lansfield, who was at the Institute at that time. One of the most vicious forms was Type A, and that was the one that showed up most often in rheumatic fever.

Children who had had rheumatic fever were on the hospital's list, so every time one of them got another attack—and recurrence was a common feature of the disease in those days—the child would be rushed right back to the hospital, where I would do an immediate throat culture and try to grow the strep. But I found that by the time they got there with their disease, the strep was gone from their throats.

It didn't make any sense. At first I thought that maybe I didn't know how to culture it, so I sought out an ear, nose and throat specialist and went through the procedure in detail to be sure I was doing it right. Then, on a hunch, we changed the timing of our studies, advising the parents on our list to bring their children into the hospital as soon as they got a sore throat, and not to wait for the rheumatic fever attack that generally ensued. I did throat cultures on those children when they arrived, and the Type A streptococcus grew easily. But as I continued the cultures over the next couple of weeks, by the time the inflammation and joint swelling appeared, the strep had gone away. We knew that the tonsils were still infected, but that was under the surface.

It dawned on me that this was the same thing that Osler had noticed with asthma. Any allergic state created by any cause—pollen, or by the germ itself—would drive the germ out of sight. The bacterial allergy of rheumatic fever had driven away the streptococcus that created the allergy. This realization was tremendously illuminating: I realized that it wasn't necessary to be able to see the germ in order to have the condition. It is reassuring to be able to culture the organism that is creating a condition, but the inability to culture it in no way means that the germ isn't still there, in hiding.

When penicillin came along and was proven to have a killing effect on the streptococcus, it wiped out rheumatic fever.

When I returned to Johns Hopkins, I began to think about the implications of this insight about allergy as it related to other diseases. I knew that undulant fever, for example, was commonly transmitted by the bodies of diseased animals to slaughterhouse workers, but that it had never been shown to be transmitted from one human to another. The reason for this had to be that the allergic response in humans was driving the brucella underground and sterilizing the surfaces in just the same way that rheumatic fever sterilized the surfaces of streptococci.

Eventually, I realized that the same process was going on in rheumatoid arthritis, and just because we couldn't see the mycoplasma, there was no reason to believe it wasn't still there, causing the trouble. That also explained the great difficulty we were having in growing mycoplasma in a culture medium. It was highly allergy-producing, it sensitized the host, and the allergic reaction was covering it up. In effect, mycoplasma planted a forest and then hid among the trees.

But we realized that this same forest was also protecting the host from an unwelcome intruder. The conventional view of allergies as a mean twist in the immune system causing something to go awry was no longer quite as valid. Nature put the allergic reaction in place in order to isolate the disease source and keep it from spreading. It happens to give symptoms, but there is a reason for it. I remembered a comment by one of my early teachers, Dr. William Tillett, who told me that in order to understand disease it was necessary to take a germ's-eye view.

For his illustration of how the germ sees things, Dr. Tillett invited me to consider why the pneumococcus germ chooses the lung as the place to live out its life, or why the meningococcus selects the meninges that surround the brain, or why the poliovirus picks one small cell in the spinal column to do its work and nowhere else, or why the typhoid bacillus chooses a small lymphoid patch in the intestinal tract from which to go out and do all its dirty work in the body. I said, "I suppose it's because those diseases find some kind of enzyme systems in those places that supports their lives, and they can't find those enzymes anywhere else."

"I think you've got it," Dr. Tillett said.

When I found that mycoplasmas had an attraction for the synovium and for the lung and the genital tract, I assumed it was because there was something present in those areas which would support them—in some cases for years. With mycoplasmas, we need further research to determine what that source of special attraction might be.

As for the significance of our understanding of the allergic state, we know that it serves a useful purpose in keeping the germ from spreading, but it doesn't stop it from producing toxins to which the body can become allergic and which then produce disease. We also know that if the treatment neutralizes those toxins that keep the germ localized—by using cortisone or too much anti-inflammatory medication—and doesn't go for their source, then all the treatment does is deprive the body of its one natural defense, letting the cat out of the bag. That process characterizes the typical course of conventional arthritis treatment: great quantities of pain-relievers, most of which are anti-inflammatory, give momentary symptomatic remission at the same time as they allow the disease to spread. And when they fail, they fail terribly.

At one time, the principal anti-inflammatory was cortisone. I recall one patient who came to me with a terrific cortisone dependency. Her previous doctors couldn't get the dosage level down, and she began to get sick from the cortisone effect, developing an ulcer in the gastrointestinal tract, hemorrhages, and other problems. The reason they couldn't lower the cortisone was that by then the cat was out of the bag and they were trying to use the same drug that had released it to block the pain produced everywhere in her body. Even to reduce her daily dose from fifty milligrams to forty-nine produced terrible pain. When she arrived at the Institute, we went for the source of the problem with intravenous tetracycline to attack the mycoplasma directly. Simply by suppressing the antigen in this manner, within three weeks we were able to reduce her cortisone requirement by 80 percent.

These days, most doctors are really afraid of cortisone, and they often go to extremes to avoid using it at all. I have never had a fear of cortisone in small doses and I frequently use it to deal with the inflammation while I attack the source of the antigen with antibiotics. The danger is not in using cortisone as a palliative, but rather in relying on it as the primary therapeutic weapon; the requirement is bound to keep mounting as the antigen, which it ignores, is allowed to increase unchecked.

The only acceptable excuse for liberating antigen in a rheumatoid arthritic is to kill its source.

To that end, we start off a typical patient with tetracycline three times a week, usually on Monday, Wednesday, and Friday. The drug is not manufactured in units less than 250 milligrams, although at one time I had it made up in

10-milligram amounts and gradually increased it to avoid the Herxheimer reaction. Nowadays we start off with the 250 milligrams, letting the Herxheimer effect occur and then treating it with symptomatic remedies.

People vary enormously in the anti-inflammatory drugs which they can use during this stage of treatment. We often start with aspirin, but we also use a wide variety of substitutes for cortisone—and sometimes small doses of the cortisone itself (one to five milligrams of prednisone a day, for example, but never more than ten and preferably none) to block the inflammatory reaction. We are careful to keep the doses of any of these drugs low enough that we don't interfere with the immune system, but rather just deal with the allergy.

An interesting thing happens to people who have a lot of regular allergies such as hay fever and skin eruptions and who start treatment for the bacterial allergy of rheumatoid arthritis: the regular allergies often get better. This points to the possibility that bacterial allergies may be one of the pacesetters for the general allergic state. I suspect that to be the case: that there is a primary allergen which in many instances comes from bacteria, and that it is added to by feathers, dust, pollen, and other irritants, and that those outside sources, long regarded as primary, may in fact be secondary.

As the treatment progresses, the doctor gradually increases the amount of antibiotic. There are lots of ways to do this: it can move up to 250 milligrams twice a day two days a week; twice a day three times a week; or a larger dosage on the original schedule of once a day three times a week. Care has to be taken not to go so high that the treatment triggers an allergic reaction; arthritics are so sensitized that they can become allergic to just about anything, including medicines that don't normally cause much allergy. The most I would prescribe orally would be 500 milligrams three times a day on Monday and Friday.

If the patient doesn't respond as well as I'd like to oral medication, I administer the drug intravenously. Recently I saw a patient who came up from Ecuador, and she had been treated with every drug available—cortisone, gold, Plaquenil, chloroquine—and had not only become refractory to each of those forms of medicine but was getting steadily and predictably worse. Moreover, it was virtually impossible to treat her with oral medicines because she had built up a resistance to practically everything. I treated her intravenously with tetracycline and a fair amount of pain-relieving anti-inflammatory medicine, and she did very well. She was not particularly exceptional; a lot of the patients we get have been so badly overmedicated that the stomach reacts to almost any medicine we put in it and we have to treat them by injection.

Regardless of how badly a patient has been sensitized to medicines, either from prior medication or from the disease itself, there is almost always some way to get around an adverse reaction until the system is back in sufficient balance to accept medication without adverse effects.

Not all of the standard treatments run out of steam after the same length of time. Gold tends to work for quite a while, often two years and sometimes longer, before it folds up. Once the patient gets sensitized to the first of these substances, however, the next ones to come along don't hold up for quite as long; either the drug loses its initial beneficial effect in a shorter time or the drug starts to produce other effects, such as skin eruptions, and treatment has to be stopped. All other things being equal, the standard drug which the patient can usually tolerate the longest is gold, followed by Plaquenil and then penicillamine. As noted repeatedly in this book, the basic problem with every one of these drugs is that each is extremely dangerous in its own right, regardless of the effects it may have on the process of sensitization; each can be lethal.

Very difficult cases of sensitization require a certain amount of persistence in seeking the right combination of antibiotic dosage and method of administration. And it is not possible to overstate the necessity for caution in the use of cortisone, which in excessive quantities can interfere with the body's defenses. The defense mechanism and the allergic mechanism are tied together in a way; an allergy is itself a form of defense and plays a role in keeping germs suppressed; on another level, the antibody seems to attach itself to the organism, making it possible for the white blood cell to become active in destroying the germ. If too much cortisone is given, that second level of defense is blocked and the purpose of the primary medicine is defeated. A small amount of an anti-inflammatory drug, sometimes even cortisone, on the other hand, suppresses the inflammatory component without blocking the basic immune mechanism, allowing the antibiotic to breach the wall around the organism and do its work.

In that connection, it has been well established that when a medicine blocks a reaction, as cortisone does, and then is stopped, the result is an explosion. When a woman goes into remission during pregnancy, it is because the body is producing extra amounts of natural cortisone to block the arthritis, and when the baby is born the mother suffers a terrible rebound flare. It is particularly difficult for an arthritic mother to have to go through this painful experience right at the time she is trying to take care of her new baby. For that reason, we often hold off on anti-inflammatory medication during the period of the pregnancy, but as soon as the mother is delivered we give it to her right away in order to avoid that flare.

The length of time patients require in treatment can vary widely, depending primarily on how long they have had the disease. In the most entrenched and recalcitrant cases, it can take up to thirty months from the beginning of therapy until the patient clearly turns the corner toward improvement, and the achievement of lasting remission can take several years.

Once the blood begins to look good, the anemia is corrected, the rheumatoid factor is down, the sedimentation and hemoglobin are where they ought to be, and the mycoplasma antibodies are beginning to peter out, I know the patient is close to remission. The antibodies are probably the key indicator; they start high, rise with the Herxheimer reaction, and then begin to fall as therapy is continued. Even if the progress toward recovery should turn downward again for a short time, the disease doesn't ever go back to the beginning, and if a situation begins to slide the physician has plenty of time to retrieve it before the patient loses any substantial ground. I always keep up the treatment until all of the blood tests look good and stay there for a reasonable length of time. In shorter-term cases—and short term doesn't necessarily mean less severe—complete remission can be achieved in less than six months.

PUBLICATIONS

Thomas McPherson Brown, M.D.

1. Tillett WS, Brown TMcP: *Epidemic meningococcus meningitis; analysis of 26 cases.* Bull Johns Hopkins Hospital 57:297–316, 1935.
2. Brown TMcP: *Protective action of sulfanilamide and anitmeningococcus serum on meningococcus infection of mice.* Bull Johns Hopkins Hospital 61:272–279, 1937.
3. Hamman L, Brown TMcP: *Subacute bacterial endocarditis.* Internat Clin 3:33–40, 1937.
4. Thomas HM Jr, and Brown TMcP: *Pulmonary emphysema complicated by hyperthyroidism.* Internat Clin 3:47–54, 1937.
5. Swift HF, Brown TMcP: *Pathogenic pleuropneumonia-like organisms from acute rheumatic exudates and tissues.* Science 89:271–272, 1939.
6. Swift HF, Brown TMcP: *Attempts to cultivate pleuropneumonia-like organisms from rheumatic exudates.* 3rd Internatl Congr Microbiol (NY 1939) Report of Proceedings 183, 1940.
7. Brown TMcP, Nunemaker JC: *Rat-bite fever with arthritis due to Streptobacillus moniliformis.* Bull Johns Hopkins Hospital 66:325, 1940.
8. Brown TMcP, Swift HF, Watson RF: *Pseudo-colonies simulating those of pleuropneumonia-like microorganisms.* J Bact 40:857–867, 1940.
9. Brown TMcP, Harvey AM: *Spontaneous hypoglycemia in "smoke" drinkers.* JAMA 117:12–15, 1941.
10. Brown TMcP, Nunemaker JC: *Rat-bite fever; review of American cases with reevaluation of etiology; report of cases.* Bull Johns Hopkins Hospital 70:201–327, 1942.
11. Brown TMcP, Hayes GS: *Isolation of microorganisms of the pleuropneumonia group from apparently pure cultures of the gonococcus.* J Bact 43:82, 1942.
12. Brown TMcP, Stifler WC Jr, Bethea WR Jr: *Early filariasis.* Bull Johns Hopkins Hospital 78:126–154, 1946.
13. Bordley JE, Brown TMcP: *Tonsillectomy in early convalescence from acute tonsillitis with prophylactic use of sulfonamides.* Ann Otol, Rhin & Laryng 55:751–753, 1946.
14. Report from Office of the Surgeon General, US Army: *History of filariasis in soldiers during World War II.* Archives of the Surgeon General, USA, World War II.
15. Report from Office of the Surgeon General, US Army: *Early filariasis. A review.* Archives of the Surgeon General, USA, World War II.
16. Brennan AJ, Brown TMcP, Warren J, Vranian G: *Syndrome characterized by generalized cutaneous eruption, chorioretinitis and eosinophilia, probably due to chronic toxoplasma infection.* Am J Med 7:431–436, 1949.
17. Brown TMcP, (L Dienes & HJ Weinberger): *Pleuropneumonia-like organisms and their possible relation to articular disease: Discussion.* Proc Seventh Int Congress of Rheumatic Diseases. In: *Rheumatic Diseases* Arth & Rheum Assoc WB Saunders Co, Philadelphia, 1952, p 407–408.
18. Brown TMcP, Wichelhausen RH, Robinson LB, Merchant WR: *The in vivo action of aureomycin on pleuropneumonia-like organisms associated with various rheumatic diseases.* J Lab Clin Med 34:1404–1410, 1949.
19. Brown TMcP, Wichelhausen RH: *Tuberculous peritonitis treated with streptomycin.* Am J Med 6:506, 1949 (Abstract).
20. Wichelhausen RH, Brown TMcP: *Tuberculous peritonitis treated with streptomycin.* Am J Med 8:421–444, 1950.
21. Brown TMcP, Merchant, WR, Wichelhausen RH, Robinson LB: *A study of the basic mechanisms in rheumatic disease.* Symposium on Cortisone and ACTH, VA Central Office, Washington DC August 1950. Published by Merck & Co, Inc, Rahway, NJ.
22. Merchant WR, Zimmerman HJ, and Brown TMcP: *Turbidimetric estimation of gamma globulin in rheumatic diseases.* Annual meeting of the Eastern Section of the American Federation for Clinical Research, Washington DC December 1950.
23. Brown TMcP, Wichelhausen RH, Merchant WR, Robinson LB: *A study of the antigen-antibody mechanism in rheumatic diseases.* Transactions Amer Clin & Climatological Assoc 62:1, 1950. Also published in Amer J Med Sci 221:618, 1951.
24. Merchant WR, Brown TMcP, Robinson LB, Wichelhausen RH: *Observations on the effect of intravenous human serum albumin in hypersensitivity reactions and various arthritic states.* (Abstract) American Society of Clinical Investigation, Atlantic City Meeting, May 1951.
25. Wichelhausen RH, Brown TMcP, Robinson LB, Merchant WR: *Pleuropneumonia-like organisms and their possible significance in collagenous diseases.* Proc. of American Rheumatism Association, Atlantic City, June 1951. Ann Rheumat Dis 10:463, 1951 (Abstract).
26. Robinson LB, Wichelhausen RH, Brown TMcP: *Sensitivity studies on human pleuropneumonia-like organisms.* J Lab Clin Med 39:290, 1952.
27. Brown TMcP: *The era of anticipatory medicine.* Med Ann of DC 23:524, 1954.
28. Brown TMcP: *The doctor-patient relationship in chronic illness.* Texas Reports on

Biol & Med 12:587, 1954.
29. Bush SW, Robinson LB, Wacker WEC, Brown TMcP: *Report of a case of collagen disease (scleroderma) in which pleuropneumonia-like organisms were isolated from an ovarian cyst.* Program of Southern Society for Clinical Research Jan 1955 (Abstract).
30. Brown TMcP: *The puzzling problem of the rheumatic diseases.* Maryland State Medical Journal 6:88–109, 1956.
31. Brown TMcP: *The rheumatic crossroads.* Postgrad Medicine, 19 (4):399–402, 1956.
32. Cooper CD, Felts WR, Brown TMcP, Wichelhausen RH: *Determination of redox activity of leukocytes as a diagnostic aid in systemic lupus erythematosus.* J Lab and Clin Med 53:457–467, 1958.
33. Clark HW, Brown TMcP, Wichelhausen RH: *Standardization of serum protein analysis by paper electrophoresis.* Federation Proceedings 17:202, 1958 (Abstract).
34. Robinson LB, Brown TMcP, Wichelhausen RH: *Studies on the effect of erythromycin and antimalarial compounds on pleuropneumonia-like organisms.* Antibiotics and Chemotherapy Vol IX:111–114, 1959.
35. Clark HW, Fowler RC, Brown TMcP: *Preparation of pleuropneumonia-like organisms for microscopic study.* J Bact 81:500–502, 1961.
36. Brown TMcP, Bush SW, Felts WR; *Rheumatoid Disease and Gout in Chapter 6 Long Term Illness.* MG Wohl (Ed) WB Saunders Co 1959.
37. Bailey JS, Clark HW, Felts WR, Fowler RC, Brown TMcP: *Antigenic properties of pleuropneumonia-like organisms from tissue cell cultures and the human genital area.* J Bact 82:542–547, 1961.
38. Clark HW, Bailey JS, Fowler RC, Brown TMcP: *Identification of Mycoplasmataceae by fluorescent antibody method.* J Bact 85:111–118, 1963.
39. Bailey JS, Clark HW, Felts WR, Brown TMcP: *Growth inhibitory properties of mycoplasma antibody.* J Bact 86:147–150, 1963.
40. Fowler RC, Coble DW, Kramer NC, Brown TMcP: *Starch gel electrophoresis of a fraction of certain of the pleuropneumonia-like group of microorganisms.* J Bact 86:1145–1151, 1963.
41. Clark HW, Bailey JS, Brown TMcP: *Determination of mycoplasma antibodies in humans.* Bacteriol Proc 64:59, 1964, M87.
42. Clark HW, Bailey JS, Brown TMcP: *New observations of mycoplasma infectivity and immunity.* Fifth Interscience Conference on Antimicrobial Agents and Chemotherapy. IVth Internat Cong of Chemotherapy, Oct 1965 (Abstract).
43. Brown TMcP, Bailey JS, Felts WR, Clark HW; *Mycoplasma antibodies in synovia.* Arth & Rheum 9:495, 1966 (Abstract).
44. Clark HW, Bailey JS, Brown TMcP: *Variations in mycoplasma antigen activity.* In *Mycoplasma Diseases Of Man.* M Sprossig and W Witzleb (Ed), Proc of the Intl Symposium, Reinhardsbrunn Castle, VEB Gustov Fischer Verlag Jena 45–58, 1969.
45. Brown TMcP, Bush SW, Felts WR: *Rheumatoid disease and gout in relation to digestive tract disorders. Chapt 66* In Gastroenterologic Medicine. M Paulson (Ed), Lea and Febiger publishers, 1969.
46. Fowler RC, Brown TMcP, Clark HW: *Mycoplasmata and bacterial L-forms in rheumatoid diseases.* In Proc Conf on the Relationship of Mycoplasma to Rheumatoid Arthritis & Related Diseases. J Decker (Ed), USPHS Pub # 1523 195–205, 1966.
47. Fowler RC, Coble DW, Kramer NC, Pai RR, Serrono BA, Brown TMcP: *Immunoelectrophoresis analyses of an aqueous fraction of some mycoplasmata and bacterial L-forms.* Ann NY Acad Sci 143:641–653, 1967.
48. Brown TMcP, Felts WR, Bush SW, Fowler RC, Oliver CH: *A systematic evaluation of arthritis and connective tissue disorders.* R&D Grant Report 1711M68C3 to SRS of the Dept of HEW, 1969.
49. Brown TMcP: *The Arthritis Story.* Reprinted from GW: The George Washington University Magazine Spring 1968 9–13.
50. Brown TMcP, Bailey JS, Clark HW, Gray WW, Clevenger AB, Heilen R: *Rheumatoid-type illness in gorilla with immunologic association of isolated mycoplasma and clinical remission following intravenous oxytetracycline therapy.* 9th Interscience Confer on Antimicrobial Agents and Chemotherapy 1969. (Abstracts)
51. Brown TMcP, Bailey JS, Clark HW, Gray CW, Clevenger AB, Heilen R: *Rheumatoid-type illness in gorilla with immunologic association of isolated mycoplasma and clinical remission following intravenous oxytetracycline therapy.* Smithsonian Inst Nat'l Zoological Park annual report 1970.
52. Brown TMcP, Clark HW, Bailey JS: *Relationship between mycoplasma antibodies and rheumatoid factors (RF).* Arth & Rheum 13:309–310, 1970.
53. Clark HW, Bailey JS, Brown TMcP: *Mycoplasma: Potential autoantigens?* X International Cong of Microbiology 92, 1970.
54. Brown TMcP, Clark HW, Bailey JS, Gray CW: *A mechanistic approach to treatment of rheumatoid-type arthritis naturally occurring in a gorilla.* Trans Amer Clin and Climatol Assn 82:227–247, 1970.
55. Brown TMcP, Felts WR, Bush SW, Oliver CH: *A study of rehabilitation potential in arthritis through programmed analysis.* R&D Grant Report BD-55079/3-02 to SRS of the Dept of HEW, 1971.
56. Clark HW, Bailey JS, Brown TMcP: *Mycoplasma variations induced by penicillin.* Bacteriol Proc 1971 (Abstract).
57. Clark HW, Brown TMcP: *Association of mycoplasma antigens with vaccines from cell cultures.* Bacteriol Proc 82 1972 (Abstract).
58. Bailey JS, Clark HW, Brown TMcP: *Char-*

acteristics of rabbit induced antibodies to human synovium and their relationship to mycoplasma. Bacteriol Proc 82, 1972 (Abstract).

59. Brown TMcP, Clark HW, Bailey JS: *Mycoplasma in pleural effusion of rheumatoid arthritis.* XIIIth International Congress of Rheumatology, Japan. Abstract 594 in Excerpta Medica 1973.
60. Clark HW, Bailey JS, Brown TMcP: *Mycoplasma antigenic and immunogenic activity.* Am Soc Microbiol Abstracts, M 35:79, 1973.
61. Brown TMcP, Clark HW, Bailey JS: *Natural occurrence of rheumatoid arthritis in great apes–a new animal model.* Proc of the Centennial Symposium on Science and Research, Zoological Society of Philadelphia 49–79, 1974.
62. Bailey JS, Clark HW, Brown TMcP Iden KI: *Radial diffusion analysis of mycoplasma desoxyribonuclease.* Am Soc Mircobiol Abstracts, 59, 1975.
63. Clark HW, Brown TMcP: *Another look at mycoplasma.* Arth & Rheum 19:649–650, 1976.
64. Clark HW, Bailey JS, Brown TMcP: *Mycoplasma-hypersensitivity reactions.* Proc Soc Gen Microbiol III: 171, 1976.
65. Brown TMcP, Clark HW, Boswell JT, Bailey JS: *The essential role of the joint scan to assess basic therapeutic gain in rheumatoid arthritis.* XIV Int'l Congr Rheum 1977. Abstract # 551, 137.
66. Clark HW, Bailey JS, Brown TMcP: *Mycoplasma hypersensitivity in rheumatoid tissues.* XIV Int'l Congr Rheum 1977. Abstract # 1107, 247.
67. Brown TMcP, Clark HW: *Rheumatoid Inflammation–Part I* Inflow 11:1–2, 1978. (See reference 65)
68. Brown TMcP, Clark HW: *Rheumatoid Inflammation–Part II* Inflow, 12:1–2, 1979. (See reference 66)
69. Brown TMcP, Clark HW, Bailey JS, Gray CW: *Rheumatoid type arthritis naturally occurring in a gorilla–a three year follow-up report of a mechanistic approach to treatment.* Proc XV Int Symp uber die Erkrankungen der Zootiere, Kolmarden, 1973, pp 357–359.
70. Brown TMcP, Clark HW, Bailey JS: *Rheumatoid arthritis in the gorilla: A study of mycoplasma-host interaction in pathogenesis and treatment.* In comparative Pathology of Zoo Animals. RJ Montali, G Migaki (Ed). Smithsonian Institution Press, 1980, pp 259–266.
71. Clark HW, Laughlin DC, Bailey JS, Brown TMcP: *Mycoplasma species and arthritis in captive elephants.* J Zoo An Med 11:3–15, 1980.
72. Brown TMcP, Clark HW, Bailey JS, Attia WM: *Comparative aspects of rheumatoid arthritis in the gorilla and man.* XV Int'l Cong of Rheumatology, 1981 (Abstract)
73. Attia WM, Clark HW, Brown TMcP: *Evaluation of lymphocyte populations and their mitogenic activity in relation to serum copper and immunoglobulin levels in rheumatoid arthritis.* Annals of Allergy, Number 1 Vol 47:99–103, 1981.
74. *Mycoplasma therapy urged as adjunct in treating RA.* Rheumatology News Vol 8, No 9, October 1981.
75. Brown TMcP, Bailey JS, Iden KI, Clark HW: *Antimycoplasma approach to the mechanism and the control of rheumatoid disease.* BBCI From: *Inflammatory Diseases and Copper.* JRJ Sorenson (Ed), The Humana Press, 1982, p 391–407.
76. Attia WM, Clark HW, Brown TMcP, Ali MK, Bellanti JA: *Inhibition of polymorphonuclear leukocyte migration by sera of patients with rheumatoid arthritis.* Annals of Allergy, Vol 48:21–24, 1982.
77. Attia WM, Shams AH, Ali MKH, Jang LW, Clark HW, Brown TMcP, Bellanti JA: *Studies of phagocytic cell functions in rheumatoid arthritis. I. Phagocytic and metabolic activities of neutrophils.* Annals of Allergy, Vol 48:279–287, 1982.
78. Attia WM, Shams AJ, Ali MKH, Land LW, Clark HW, Brown TMcP Bellanti JA: *Studies of phagocytic functions in rheumatoid arthritis. II Effects of serum factors on phagocytic and metabolic activities of neutrophils.* Annals of Allergy, 48:266–279, 1982.
79. Clark HW, Bailey JS, Brown TMcP: *Properties supporting the role of mycoplasmas in rheumatoid arthritis.* Reviews of Infectious Diseases. Vol. 4:S238, 1982. (Abstract)
80. Bailey JS, Clark HW, Brown TMcP, Iden KI: *Inhibitory effects of copper on mycoplasma.* Reviews of Infectious Diseases. Vol 4:S238, 1982. (Abstract)
81. Brown TMcP: *Support of funding mycoplasma research toward the cause of arthritis.* Congressional Record Vol 128:E1447, 1982.
82. Brown TMcP: *The antimycoplasma treatment program for arthritis should be investigated by the NIH.* Congr Record Vol. 129:E2561, 1983.
83. Clark HW, Brown TMcP: *The antimycoplasma approach to the treatment of rheumatoid arthritis.* Report to U.S. House of Representatives Subcommittee for Appropriations for 1984, in Hearings Part 9, 714–741, 1983.
84. Brown TMcP, Novak JW, Hockberg MC, et al: *Antibiotic therapy of rheumatoid arthritis: An observational cohort study of 98 patients with 451 patient-years of follow-up.* XVI International Congress of Rheumatology, 1985.
85. Bailey JS, Clark HW, Brown TMcP: *Superoxide as an Agent of Toxic Potential for Mycoplasmas.* 85th Meeting, ASM, 1985.
86. Bailey JS, Clark HW, Brown TMcP, Iden I: *Profile of a Mycoplasma Isolate from Rheumatoid Synovium,* 86th Meeting, ASM, 1986.

INDEX